making beaded
fashion jewellery

Natalie Leon

making beaded fashion jewellery

Natalie Leon

First published in Great Britain in 2008
A & C Black Publishers Limited
38 Soho Square
London W1D 3HB
www.acblack.com

ISBN: 978-0-7136-8400-1

CIP Catalogue records for this book are available from the British Library and the U.S. Library of Congress.

Book design: Sally Fullam
Cover design: Sutchinda Rangsi Thompson
Photography: Dan Byrne
Commissioning Editor: Susan Kelly
Managing Editor: Sophie Page

Printed and bound in China

This book is produced using paper that is made from wood grown in managed, sustainable forests. It is natural, renewable and
recyclable. The logging and manufacturing processes conform to the environmental regulations of the country of origin.

The author and publisher cannot accept any liability for the use or misuse of any materials or equipment mentioned in this
book. Always read any product and equipment instructions and take any necessary precautions.

contents

getting started

For all of you who are new to beading, I hope you find this book useful and can constantly refer back to it, even after you've completed all the projects. I've tried to include all the things I wish someone had told me about when I started beading. The stockists list at the back of this book will help you find great beads no matter where you are. The Bead Society of Great Britain and their events and newsletters are a great resource and opportunity to meet other beaders.

Welcome to the wonderful world of beading. The step by step projects in this book will help get you started and most of these projects can be completed in under an hour. Once you start buying beads and making your own jewellery you'll find you can't stop. And why would you want to? Now you can make a new piece of jewellery every time a new trend comes out or whenever you buy a new outfit. Every birthday and Christmas present you give will be extra special because they'll be handmade and unique. You're bound to fall in love with one kind of bead in particular, for me its vintage beads and

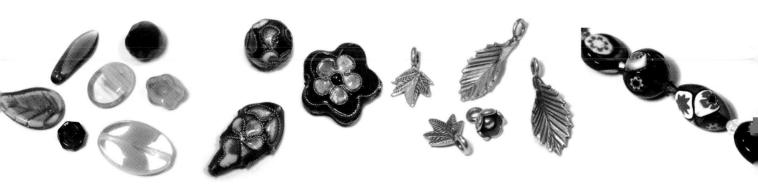

Czech Glass Beads   **Cloisonné Beads from China**   **Hill Tribe silver charms from Thailand**   **Vintage Millefiori Beads from Italy**

the struggle to find them is part of the fun. Here are some examples of just a few of the many kinds of beads for you to fall for....

Beads are measured in millimetres, and bead strands are measured in inches. Having a meter steel ruler to hand makes cutting lengths of chain and checking bead sizes much easier. Standard necklace lengths are 16, 18 and 24 inches. This chart will tell you how many beads you will need for your necklace depending on its length and the sizes of the beads you are using.

Beads to a strand

Bead Size	16 inch	18 inch	24 inch
4mm	100	112	153
6mm	68	76	100
8mm	50	56	76
10mm	40	45	61

Beads come in all shapes and sizes; here are some examples of common gemstone beads to show the many different shapes you will come across.

Seed Beads

These tiny beads come in a variety of styles, sizes and colours, including metallic and AB (Aurora Borealis) finishes. You will find them sold by size in bead shops, the larger the number the smaller the bead. Sizes 6" and 11" are the most common. Sizes 6"s make excellent spacers to be used in-between more expensive accent beads. Size 11"s are best suited to bead weaving.

Delicas Irregular cylinders, shaped like a square, with a large hole.
Bugles long narrow tubes shapes.

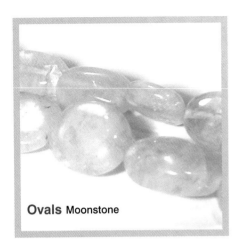

Ovals Moonstone

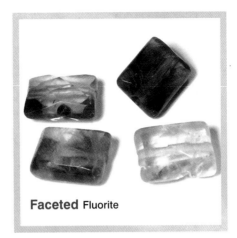

Faceted Fluorite

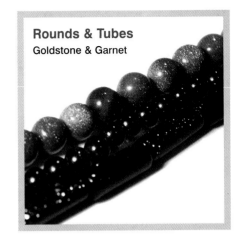

Rounds & Tubes
Goldstone & Garnet

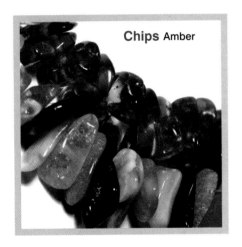

Chips Amber

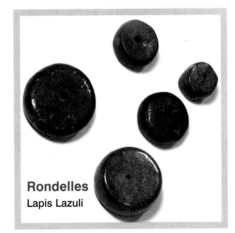

Rondelles
Lapis Lazuli

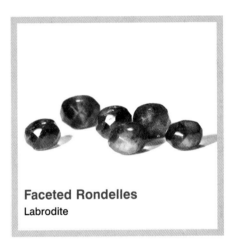

Faceted Rondelles
Labrodite

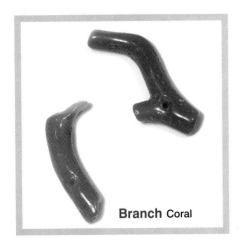

Branch Coral

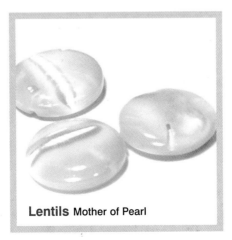

Lentils Mother of Pearl

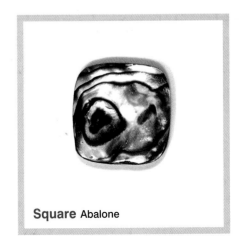

Square Abalone

Stringing materials

Tigertail is a fine steel cable coated with nylon which doesn't need to be threaded with a needle because it's very stiff. The problem with this is that it does not knot well and kinks very easily. Instead why not try two of my favourite modern alternatives that are more supple and kink resistant.

Softflex beading wire is a fantastic product that drapes beautifully and is strong. It is constructed of either 21 or 49 micro woven, stainless steel wires, braided together and then nylon coated. Unlike elastic which dries out, becomes brittle and eventually snaps. Softflex doesn't need to be knotted in-between beads like thread or cord. You can space beads out using tiny seed beads in-between larger beads or use crimps. When you're leaving spaces try experimenting with the colours available. Softflex comes in different thicknesses and colours for different projects. If you're using pearls or other beads with a small hole try the 0.14", for crystals and glass beads there's 0.19", but if you're making something with heavy semi-precious stone beads try something thicker like 0.24".

Beadalon is another great beading wire. Like Softflex it is made from several fine wires twisted together then coated with nylon, so it can also be finished with crimps. Beadalon comes in 3 different thicknesses and a huge variety of colours including: gold, silver, bronze, black, pink, red, blue, green, and purple.

The 9 strand is a good basic to have in your bead box. It's perfect to start experimenting with it, because its affordable and comes in all the available colours.

The 19 strand wire is ideal for beginners. It is more flexible than the 9 strand but still affordable and is also available in all the colours listed above.

The 49 strand is best suited to professional designers because it offers the most strength and flexibility. It is available in the metallic colours.

There are 4 main formulas for stringing beads; you can see examples in this image.
1) Symmetrical   2) Random
3) Graduated   4) Repeating

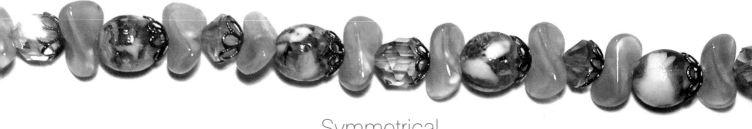

Symmetrical

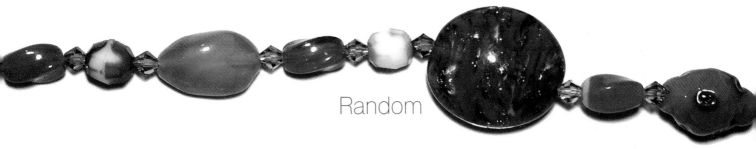

Random

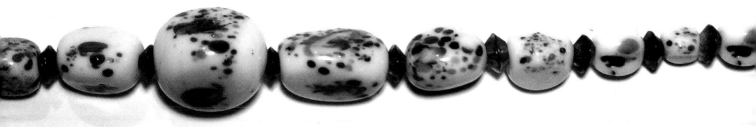

Graduated

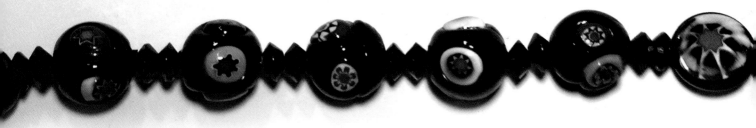

Repeating

13

basics

These 3 simple techniques are the basis for all the beading projects in this book. Once you master them you will be able to create your own designs with ease.

TECHNIQUE 1 Making plain loops

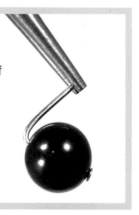

1 Thread bead onto head or eye pin. Cut off excess with wire cutters, leaving 1cm. The more wire you leave the larger your loop will be.

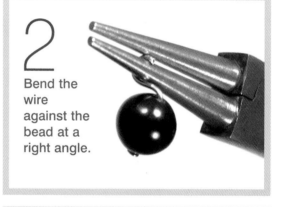

2 Bend the wire against the bead at a right angle.

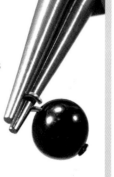

3 Grip the end of the wire using round nose pliers, and press downwards lightly as you rotate the pliers to form the loop, keep turning to close the loop.

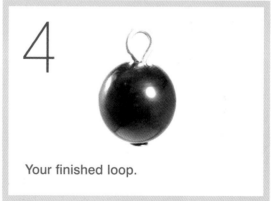

4 Your finished loop.

2 Making wrapped loops

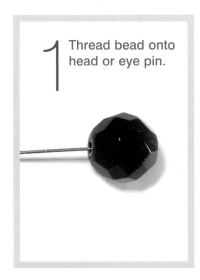

1 Thread bead onto head or eye pin.

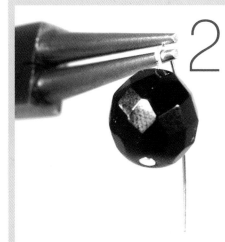

2 Grip the end of the wire nearest to the bead tightly using round nose pliers, and press downwards lightly as you rotate the pliers to create the beginning of your loop.

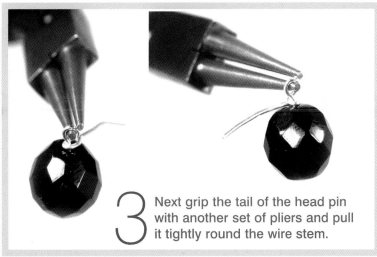

3 Next grip the tail of the head pin with another set of pliers and pull it tightly round the wire stem.

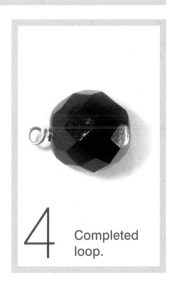

4 Completed loop.

Wrapping a Briolette (or any top drilled bead)

For wire wrapping you will need beading wire. This comes in many thicknesses and varying degrees of softness, but to start wire wrapping invest in some copper based beading wire which is easy to work with.

1 Cut an 8cm piece of wire and center your bead on it.

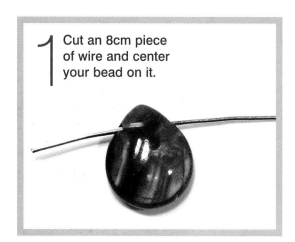

2 Carefully bend each end of the wire upwards so that they cross each other to create an X.

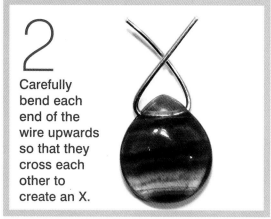

3 Take the end of right hand wire and pull it downwards diagonally across the other wire.

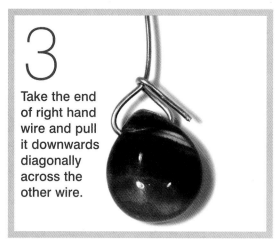

4 Still holding this wire pull it around the wire stem and trim the excess.

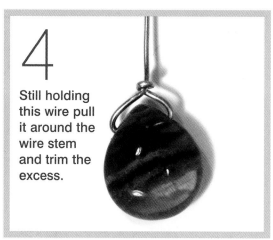

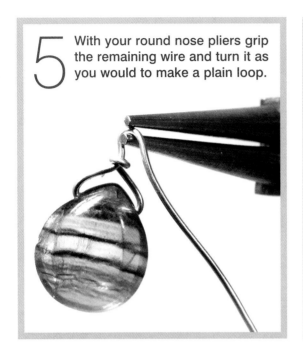

5 With your round nose pliers grip the remaining wire and turn it as you would to make a plain loop.

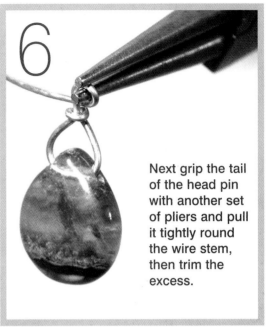

6 Next grip the tail of the head pin with another set of pliers and pull it tightly round the wire stem, then trim the excess.

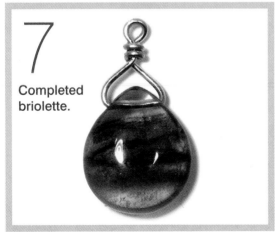

7 Completed briolette.

useful tools & findings

Pliers & Wire Cutters

Three types of pliers are commonly used in jewellery making.

Round nose pliers To make loops.
Wire cutters To trim head/eye pins, wires and threads.
Crimping pliers To crush crimp beads to finish piece.

When working with wire you may also find chain-nose pliers helpful to allow you to grip the wire more easily. These pliers are flat in the middle but round on the outside.

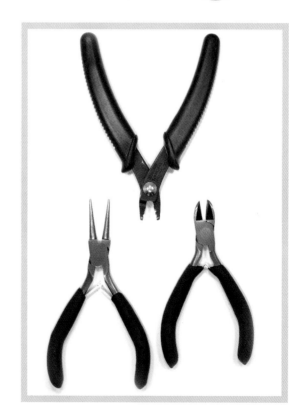

Bead Board

An inexpensive but essential item, having a bead board will make your life so much easier. You can use the board to lay out your designs before you thread them, and leave them safely while you work on other things. It has space for more than one project at a time. Whilst you're working on a piece you can also put a selection of the beads you're using in the handy trays to add beads to your design or make matching pieces later. Another option instead of a bead board is a handy bead mat; it is made of micro fibres that keep will your beads from rolling away.

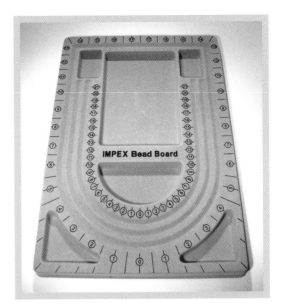

Bead Awl

This tool is helpful when you find a bead that has been coated with a finish but the hole is covered. Simply pierce through the hole with the bead awl. While this is a useful and handy tool it is also very sharp so it is not recommended for younger beaders.

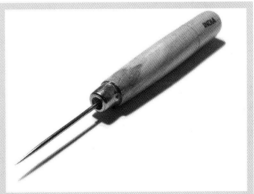

Bead Reamer

Like a tiny drill this tool is designed to make the holes in pearls and other gemstone beads slightly larger for threading.

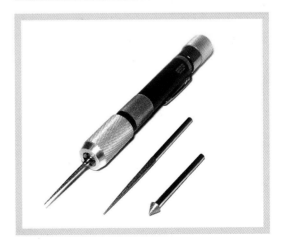

1. 2. 3. 4.

Findings

Clasps

Column one shows just some of the many clasps now widely available. These will enable you to open and close your bracelet and necklaces securely. At the top are multi-strand clasps, for five and three strand necklaces or bracelets. The next type are basic Lobster claw and Toggle clasps which are available in a variety of unique designs. At the bottom of column one are "S" clasps and a selection of antique and vintage clasps, decorated with rhinestones. All of these clasps are available in sterling silver, silver plated, gold plated, gold filled and base metal. Every clasp has a loop and the more strands the more loops the clasp will have.

Connectors & Reducers

In column two there are vintage and modern findings that allow you to make three rows into one, these are called reducers or connectors. These findings can also be used to make beautiful dangling earrings.

Earring Findings

At the bottom of column two are beadable earring hoops, which can be opened to allow you to add beads onto the hoop. Column three shows some of the findings used to make chandelier style earrings, as well as basic earring hooks and fancy Bali silver earring hooks. At the bottom are earring posts with a loop for a drop. Earring findings with open loops that are not soldered are best to use for your first projects. Later once you are more confident you will be able to design earrings that don't need an open loop.

Headpins & Eye Pins

These are essential items which you will use in every piece of jewellery you make. They are often sold in packs of 100 and whilst that may seem like a lot you will use them up quickly. An eye pin has a loop or eye at the end of it, a head pin looks like a thin nail.

Jump Rings

These come in every size and are usually either wire ovals or circles, but all are split somewhere to use them you have to open them. They are used to connect things like charms to a bracelet. Depending on your projects you may need a large one or a more delicate less visible one. To begin with buy open unsoldered jump rings that you can easily open and close. Try to resist the temptation to pull the jump ring apart by pulling one side of the ring upwards, this will only miss-shape it. Instead grasp the ring between two sets of pliers and pull each horizontally, so you are working one side slightly forward and the other side slightly back in the opposite direction.

Spacers, Bails & Bead Caps

Spacers are used in between beads, these are Bali silver spacers which can be plain and round or very ornate and shaped like stars or flowers.

Bails are glued onto things you want to use without a hole such as shells, pebbles, crystals and gemstones, which allows you to attach them to your piece using the loop on the bail.

Bead caps hide the bead holes, and are often used to add a decorative touch to a basic bead.

Crimps

Crimps are tiny little beads that once crushed (or crimped) will grip tightly onto whatever is inside them. They are used to secure the ends of necklace and bracelets made from tigertail or wire. Using them is easy, just string two crimps onto the end of your wire, then add the clasp. Loop the wire back through the crimps, which creates a loop around the clasp. Then for added security thread the wire back through two or three extra beads. Make sure the crimp beads are pushed right up against the clasp and there is very little bare wire, then crush the crimps using your crimping pliers, and trim any excess wire.

precious metals

W hen you first start beading you will probably be using plated findings, before you move on to more expensive sterling silver findings. To explain the differences here are a few definitions.

Gold

Gold is measured in karats; this tells you the quantity of gold in an alloy, pure gold is 24kt. Standard karats that you may come across 10kt, 14kt, 18kt, 22kt. So a piece that is 10kt gold has only 10/24 parts gold, whereas a 22kt piece has 22/24 parts gold. The higher the karat the more gold there is in the piece, and the finer it is.

Gold Filled

There is approximately 50-100 times more gold in a gold filled item, than gold plate. Gold filled items are often marked to show the karat of gold used e.g. 1/20 12kt GF. By definition, an item that is stamped GF, must have a minimum layer of karat gold, that is equal to at least 1/20 the weight of the total item. Gold filled items can last up to 30 years without signs of wear.

Gold plated

A layer of gold applied to base metal, by electroplating. This is usually a very thin layer, which will wear down and become discoloured. Most bead shops sell gold/silver plated findings and they are easy to work with and economical when you first get started beading.

Goldtone

Gold coloured metal that may be electro-plated, but it is not real gold so it cannot be measured in karats.

Vermeil

A layer of gold which has been electroplated over sterling silver. For something to be called vermeil, the gold has to be at least 10-karat and the surface coating must be at least 1.5 micrometers thick.

Sterling Silver

The legal definition for sterling silver is an alloy of silver containing 92.5% pure silver and 7.5% other metals, usually copper. Hallmarked 925.

Silver Plate

A layer of silver applied to base metal, by electroplating. This is usually a very thin layer, which will wear down quickly, and become discoloured over time.

a guide to choosing
& using your wire

When you first start working with wire it can be a bit confusing, trying to figure out which gauge and what kind of wire you need for what you want to make. Hopefully, this will make it a lot easier. Just remember the smaller the gauge the thicker the wire. Here is a list of the standard gauges and their uses.

16 gauge   A very heavy and thick wire. Use with heavy duty tools.
            Uses: Wire sculpture, bracelet bases, unsupported shapes, neck wires.

18 gauge   Medium thick wire.
            Uses: Wine charms, clasps, wire wrapping beads with large holes,
            chain making.

20 gauge   Medium wire. Most base metal headpins and ear wires are made from
            20-gauge wire.
            Uses: A good all-purpose wire for making ear wires, headpins, and small
            wire clasps. Good for wire wrapping most glass beads and eye pins.

22 gauge   Medium thin wire. This gauge is ideal to use when 20-gauge is just a bit
            too thick.
            Uses: Wire wrapping beads like Swarovski Crystals or semi-precious beads.

24 gauge   Thin wire. Nylon wire straightening pliers are recommended for this wire, which easily kinks.
Uses: Wire wrapping smaller crystals, semi-precious beads, and freshwater pearls to chain.

26 gauge   Very thin wire. In order for this wire to maintain a loop, loops must be wire wrapped closed. Because of the delicacy of this wire you should use tools with very fine tips. To repair kinks, nylon wire straightening pliers are recommended.
Uses: Wire wrapping beads to tiaras and in wire projects where 24-gauge wire is just a bit too heavy for the beads. Wire stitching, embroidery, and seed bead projects.

28-34 gauge   Extremely fine wire. This delicate wire, prone to kinking, should be used with nylon wire, straightening pliers and tools with very fine tips.
Uses: This wire is perfect for wire weaving, crocheting and free form wire wrapping using small beads.

Wire Hardness

Always practise first with the cheaper brass or copper based wires. Precious metal wires are made in two metals, gold filled and sterling silver. They come in four shapes: round, half round, square and twisted. Choosing the shape of the wire depends on what project you need it for. Precious metal wires come in three hardnesses:

Dead Soft Wire   This is extremely flexible and can be bent easily. However, it does not retain its shape, especially when bearing a large amount of weight/pressure.

Half Hard Wire   Whilst still flexible this wire is less likely to lose its shape under weight and pressure.

Full Hard Wire   A strong wire that keeps its shape and is excellent for clasps. Although it is not suitable for more intricate designs that require more malleability.

basic
butterfly
earrings

a

b

c

YOU WILL NEED

Headpins

4mm Czech glass beads

6mm Czech glass beads

15mm Chinese Cloisonné butterfly beads

A pair of earrings wires

1 Thread 6mm bead, Butterfly bead, and 4mm bead onto head pin. See pictures A-C.

2 Trim head pin and make loop. (See making plain loops in Basics section.)

3 Open earring wire loop and attach earrings wire/hook.

4 Finished earrings. See picture D.

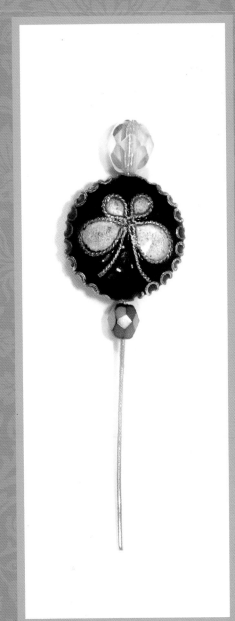

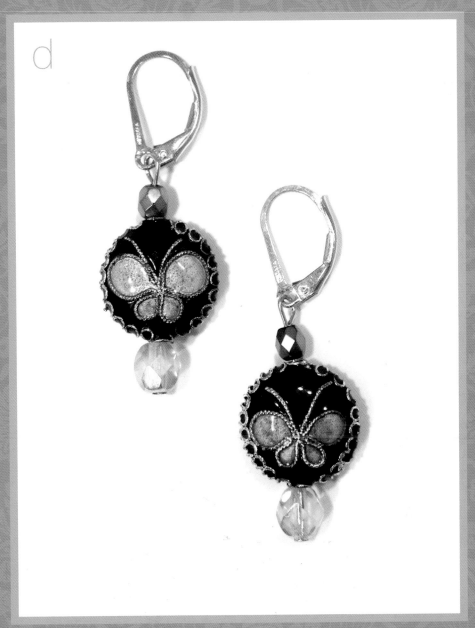

d

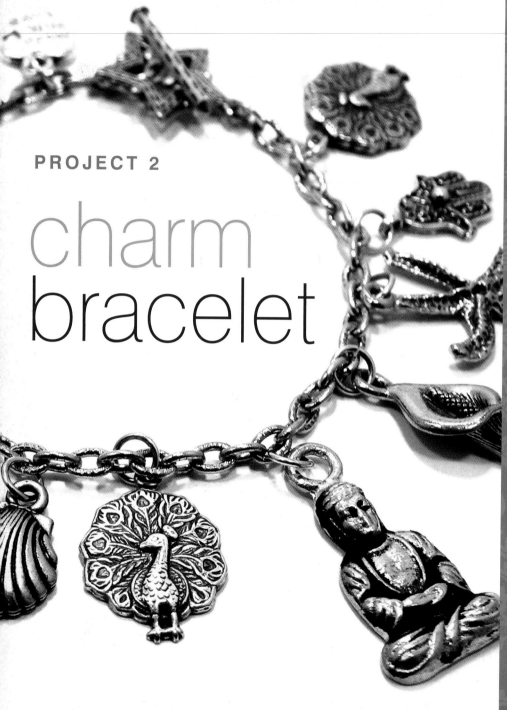

PROJECT 2

charm bracelet

1 Measure your wrist with a tape measure; leave a little excess for comfort, then using that measurement cut a length of chain to fit your wrist.

2 Using the instructions in the Findings section, open a jump ring and attach the bar from your toggle clasp. See picture A.

3 One by one open and close each jump ring to add your charms. See pictures B and C.

4 Keep adding charms till you are happy with the number of charms on your bracelet.

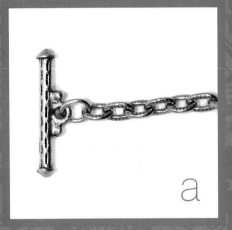

a

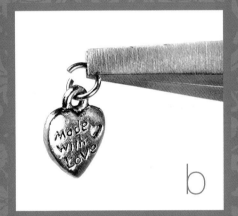

b

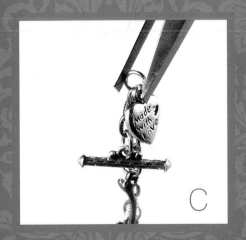

c

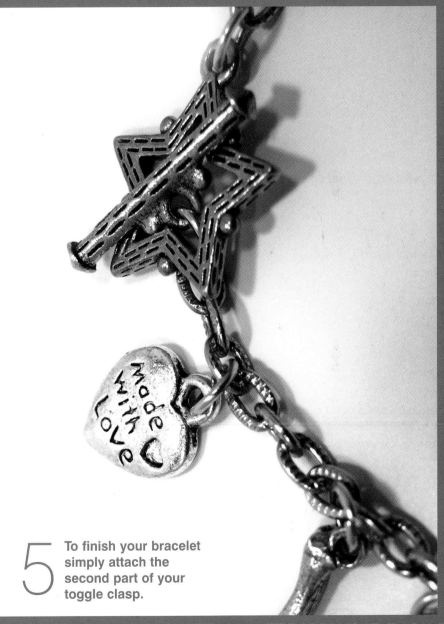

5 To finish your bracelet simply attach the second part of your toggle clasp.

step-by-step

YOU WILL NEED

4mm Swarovski crystals

6mm Swarovski crystals

Head pins

Pair of lever back earring findings

Chain

12mm Czech glass window beads

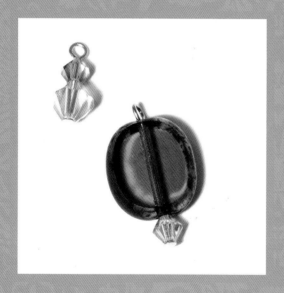

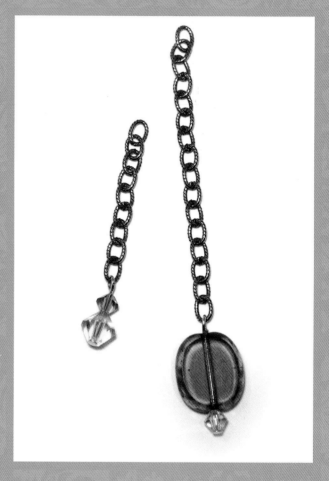

1 Make two sets of drops using your selection of Czech and Swarovski beads and eye pins. They don't have to match but try to alternate the colours and sizes for a more striking combination.

2 Cut two different lengths of chain, one 1cm longer than the other and attach them by simply opening the loops of your drops.

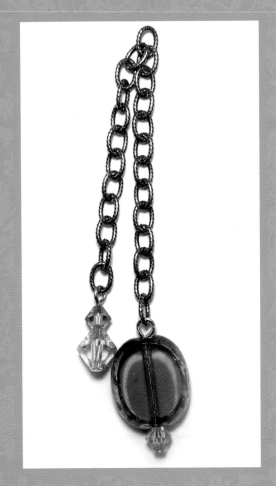

3 To attach these two chains to each other just open the top link of the chain like a jump ring and link the other chain through it.

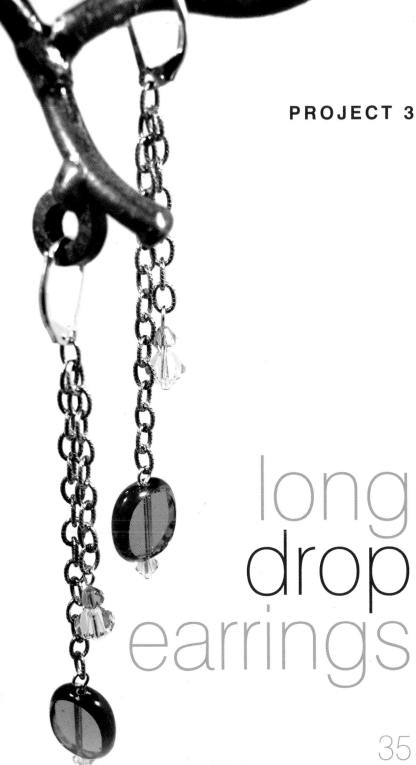

long drop earrings

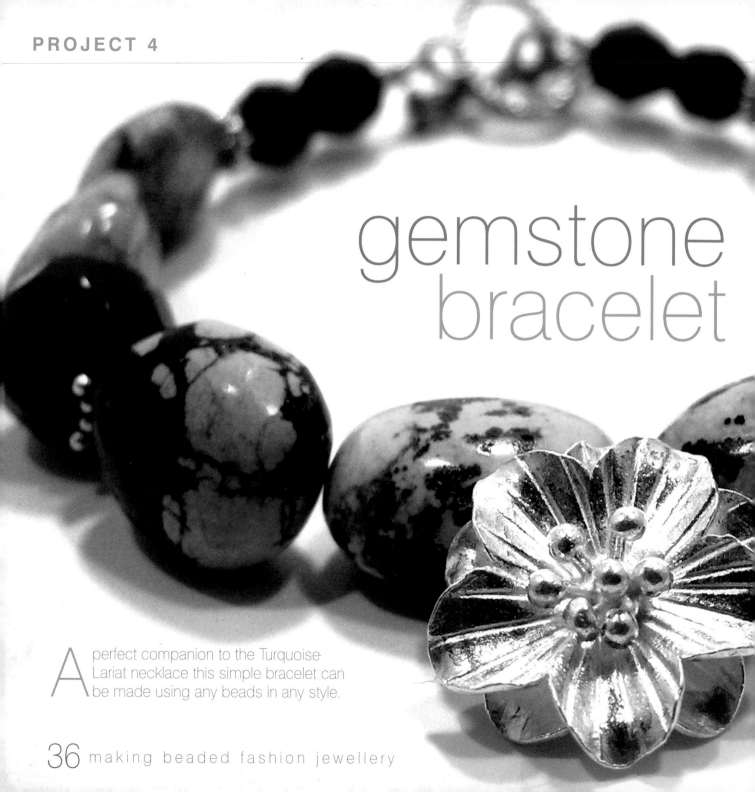

gemstone
bracelet

A perfect companion to the Turquoise Lariat necklace this simple bracelet can be made using any beads in any style.

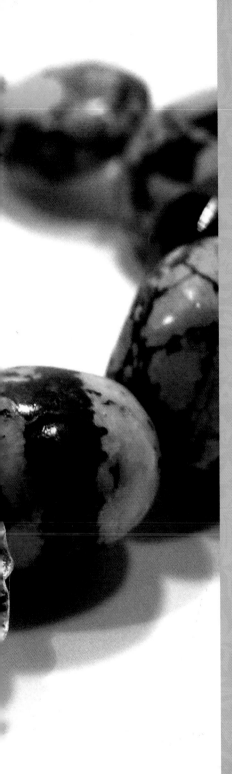

step-by-step

1 Cut a length of wire, measure your wrist and give yourself a little extra for a comfortable fit, then add an extra 3cm at each end. This allows you to thread the beads onto the wire more easily and later when you use crimps to double back for added strength and security.

2 Start stringing your beads on the thread. Look at your design, how do the beads look sitting next to one another? If you're not happy it's easy to take a few beads off and reorganise them.

YOU WILL NEED

Beadalon or Softflex beading wire

Toggle clasp

Bali silver spacers

Hill tribe Silver flower pendant

Turquoise nuggets

Black Czech glass beads in 12mm and 6mm

Crimps

Crimping pliers

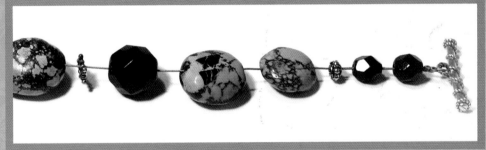

3 Once you are happy with your design, thread two crimp beads onto either end. (Using two gives you added security that your bracelet will not snap or come undone, especially when you are learning how to use crimps for the first time.)

4 Finished bracelet.

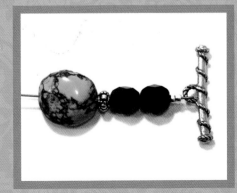

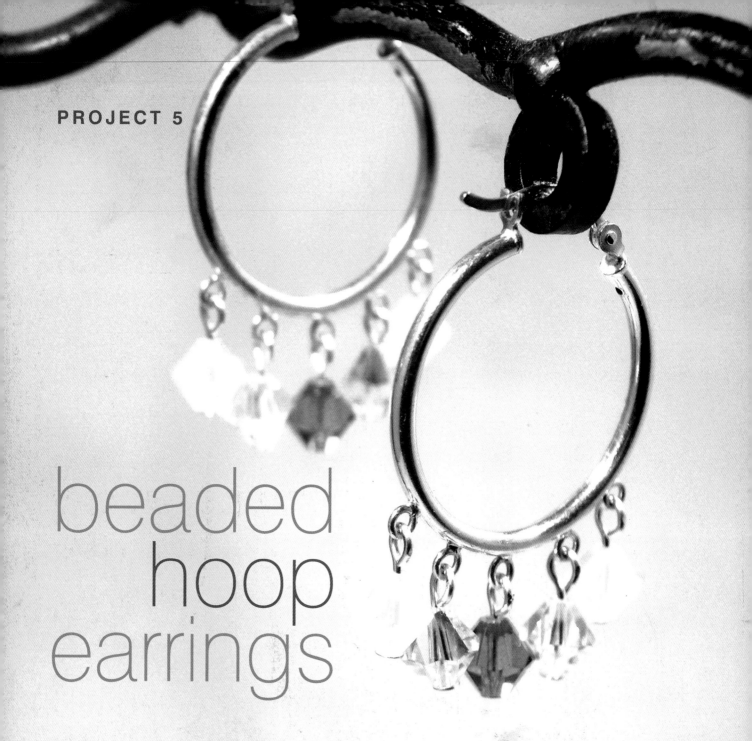

beaded
hoop
earrings

step-by-step

YOU WILL NEED

6mm Swarovski crystal beads

Head pins

Hoop earring findings with soldered loops

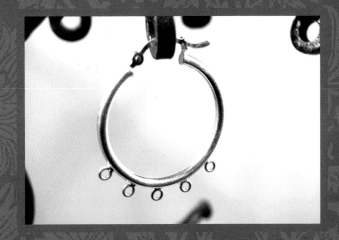

1 Start with a pair of beaded hoop findings with earring wires already attached.

2 Create a drop by putting a Swarovski crystal on a head pin and making a loop.

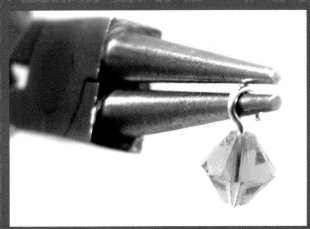

3 Add more crystals until you have used all the available loops. Then repeat on the other finding. If you prefer a more dainty look, try using two 4mm crystals on each loop instead of one 6mm crystal.

4 Completed earrings.

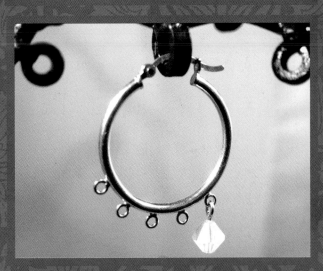

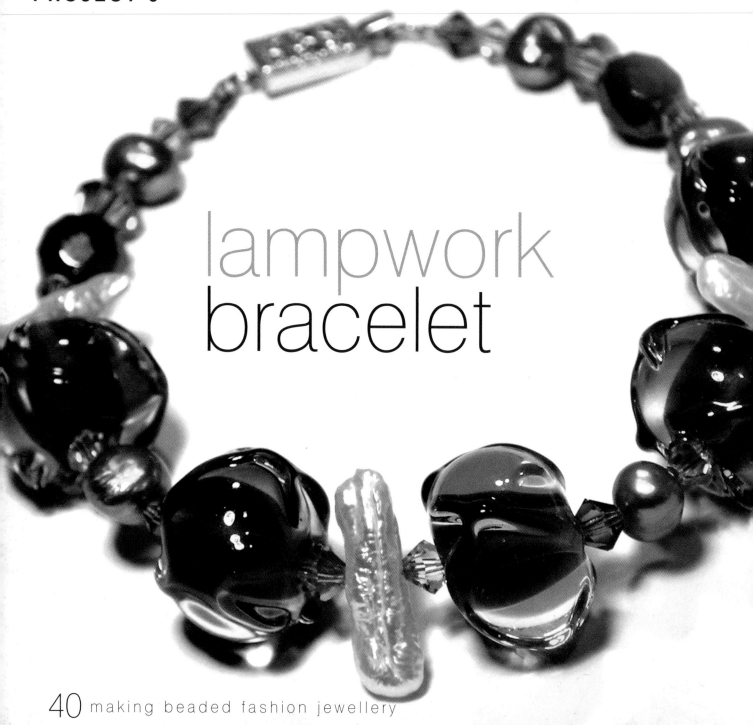

lampwork
bracelet

step-by-step

These spectacular beads were handmade especially for this book by Lampwork artist Emma Ralph. You can buy Emma's fantastic beads from her website, the details are in the stockists pages.

YOU WILL NEED

Lampwork beads

Biwa pearls

Freshwater pearls

Beading wire

Clasp

Crimps

Crimping pliers

4mm Swarovski crystals

6mm Swarovski crystals

6mm Czech glass beads

1 First thread your design onto the beading wire. Leave 3cm extra on each end, like you did in project 4. Make sure to put crystals and Czech glass beads at each end so that you can thread the beading wire back through at the end. Use pearls as accents in-between the lampwork beads.

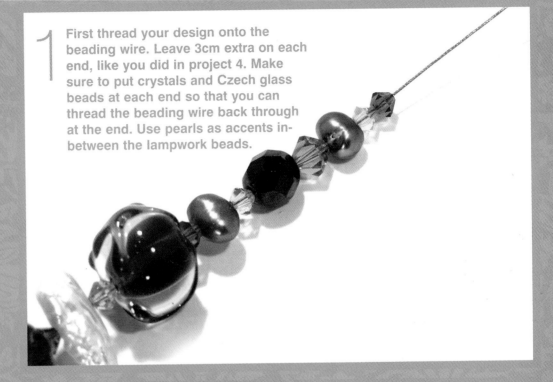

2 Check you're happy with your design.

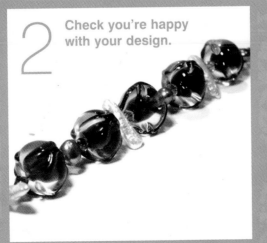

3 Add two crimps to each end of the bracelet and thread back through the clasp and three extra beads for security, then using wire cutters cut off the excess wire.

step-by-step

YOU WILL NEED

A kilt pin

Chain

Metal star beads

Abalone square beads

8mm Czech glass beads

6mm Cats eye beads

6mm Czech glass beads

Czech glass drops beads

Eye pins

Head pins

1 Start with your kilt pin; this is what they look like.

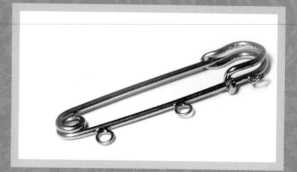

2 Cut two pieces of chain one 3cm longer than the other. Make your Abalone bead and one of your star beads into a link by putting it onto an eye pin and make another link at the opposite end. To attach the chain simply open the link like you would open a jump ring (see Findings page for a reminder).

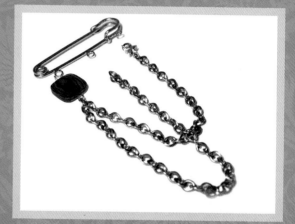

3 Start making drops with the 6mm, 8mm and teardrop Czech glass and Cats eye beads and add them to the bottom of your links. (See the Basics page for making plain loops.)

4 Keep adding beads until you have a small cluster on the right under the star and a larger cluster underneath the Abalone bead.

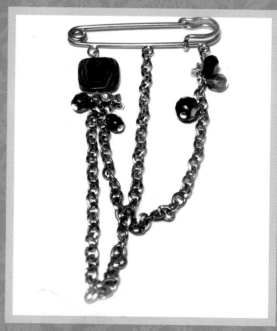

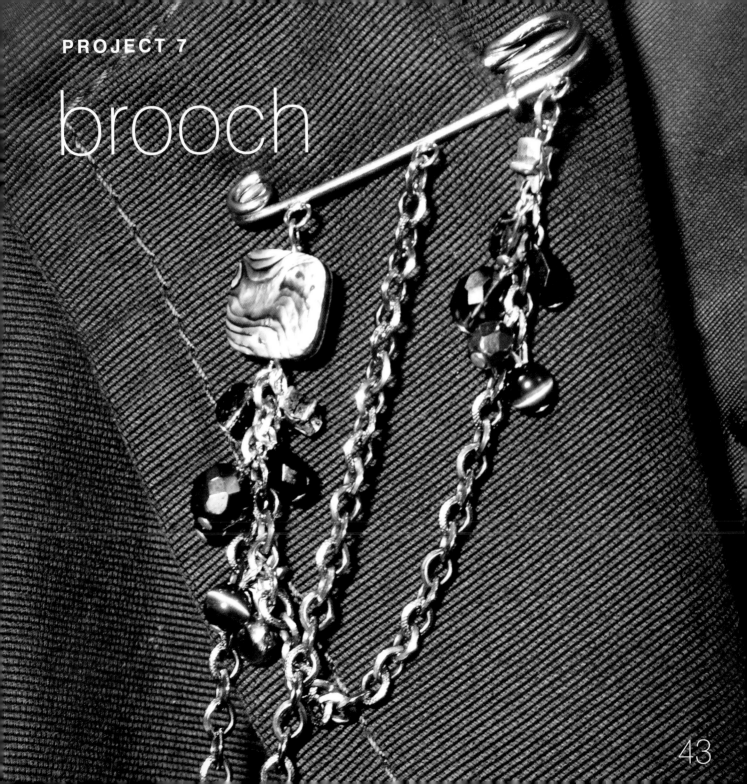

brooch

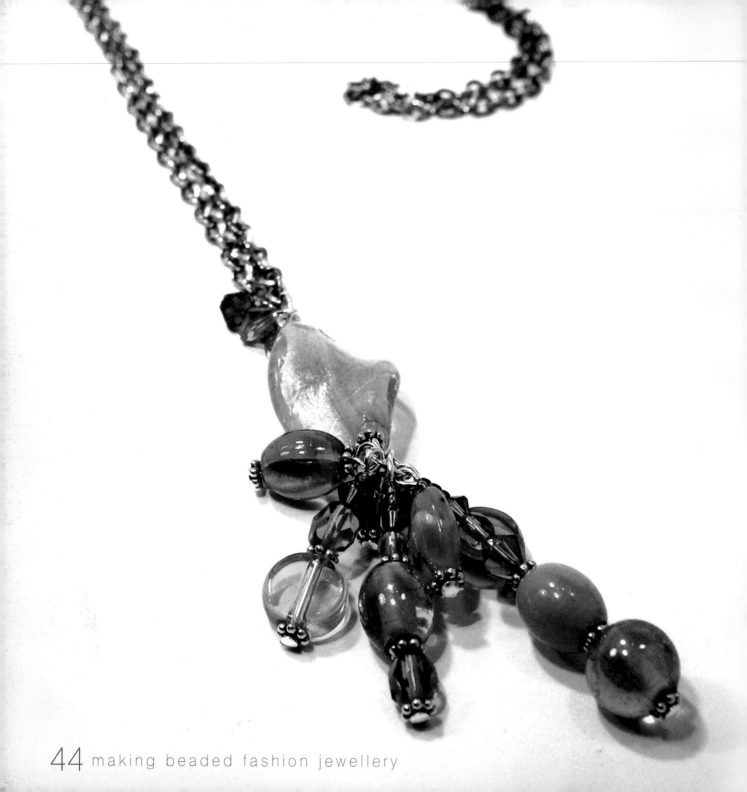

extra long chain necklace with beads

This trendy style of necklace is great over a long t-shirt or smock dress.

YOU WILL NEED

A Focal bead*

24 inches of chain

Head pins

Eye pins

Jump rings

Bali silver spacers

Size 11" seed beads

4mm glass beads

6mm glass beads

8mm glass beads

10mm glass beads

4mm Swarovski crystal beads

6mm Swarovski crystal beads

*I chose a Venetian glass focal bead available from www.beadsbydesign.co.uk.

You will find a great selection of Swarovski crystals for you to choose from at www.beadsbyyvonne.co.uk.

step-by-step

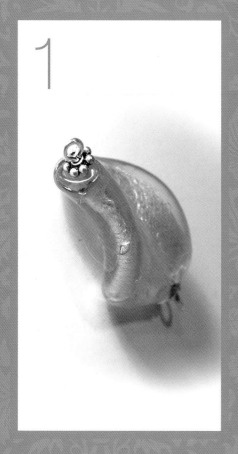

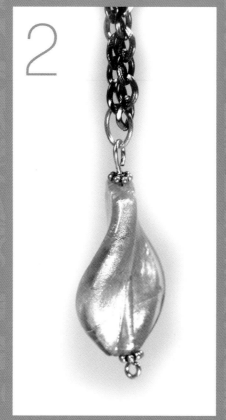

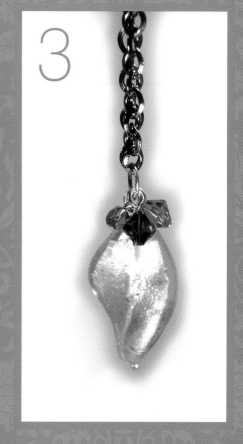

Make your focal bead into a pendant by putting a spacer at each end on an eye pin, and making a loop.

Now open your jump ring and attach the focal to both ends of your chain.

Make three small 4mm drops using your Swarovski crystals and one 6mm drop, and attach them to the jump ring at the top of your pendant.

4

To make the
beaded tassel:
make the longest
drop first.

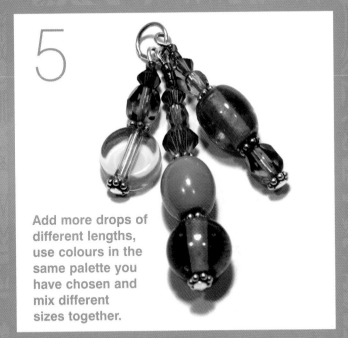

5

Add more drops of
different lengths,
use colours in the
same palette you
have chosen and
mix different
sizes together.

6

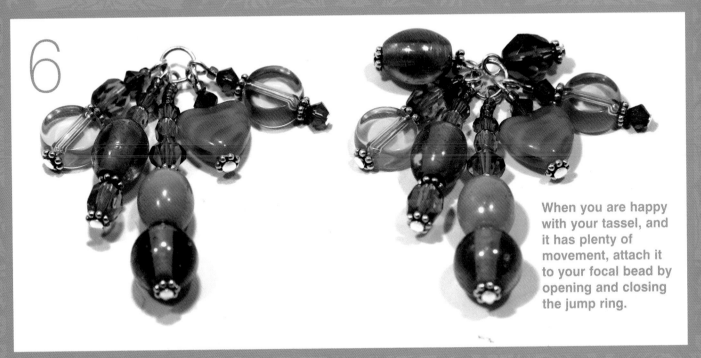

When you are happy
with your tassel, and
it has plenty of
movement, attach it
to your focal bead by
opening and closing
the jump ring.

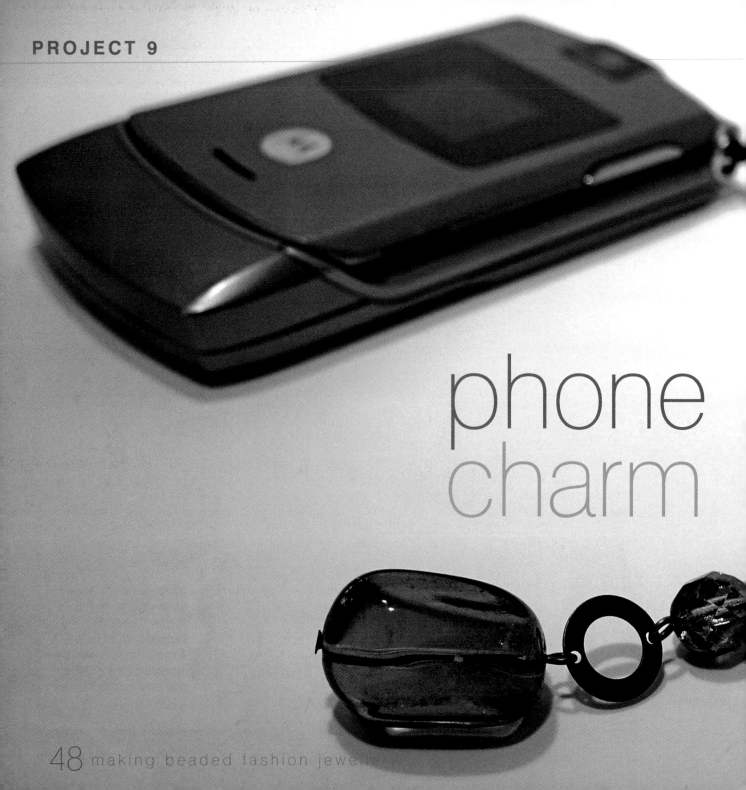

phone
charm

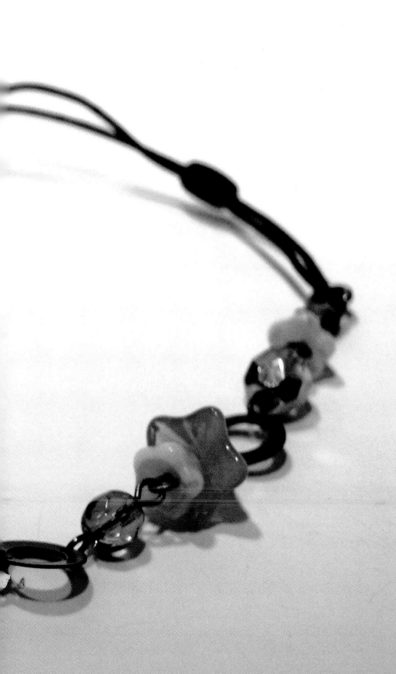

YOU WILL NEED

Decorative links

2 sizes of Czech glass flowers

8mm Czech glass beads

6mm Czech glass beads

Eye pins

Head pins

Larger Focal bead for end of charm 12-18mm

Lobster claw clasp

*These fabulous bronze colour decorative links are available from RegalCrafts; you can find their information in the stockist's pages.

step-by-step

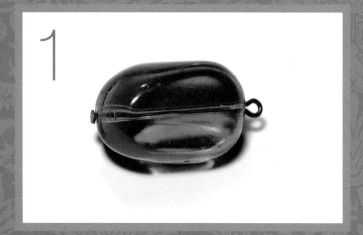

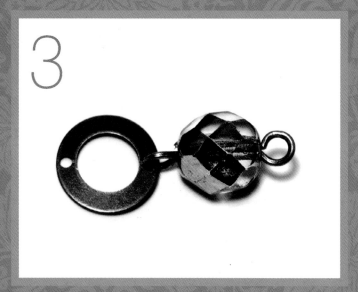

1 Make your focal bead into a drop using a head pin and making a loop.

2 Instead of using jump rings try experimenting with these great decorative links.

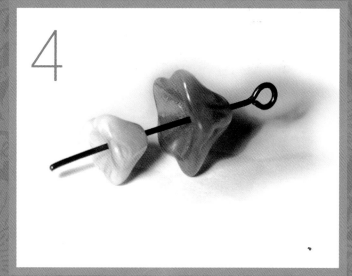

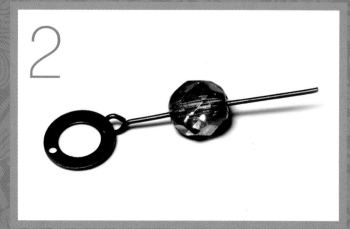

3 Make individual beaded links by adding the 6mm and 8mm beads onto your eye pins and making another loop.

4 Making the fuchsia flower drop is easy, just thread the smaller flower inside the larger one.

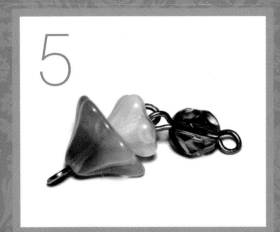

5

Your charm is ready.

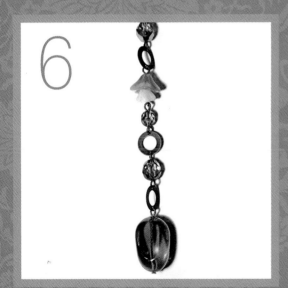

6

Open the top link of your charm to add the lobster claw clasp which you can use to attach to your phone, and change charms whenever you want.

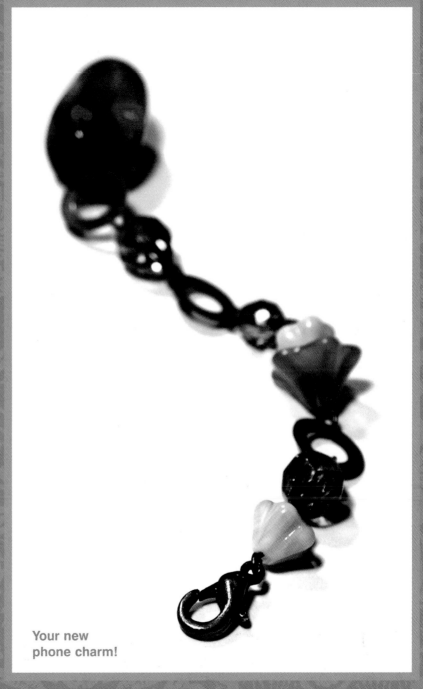

Your new
phone charm!

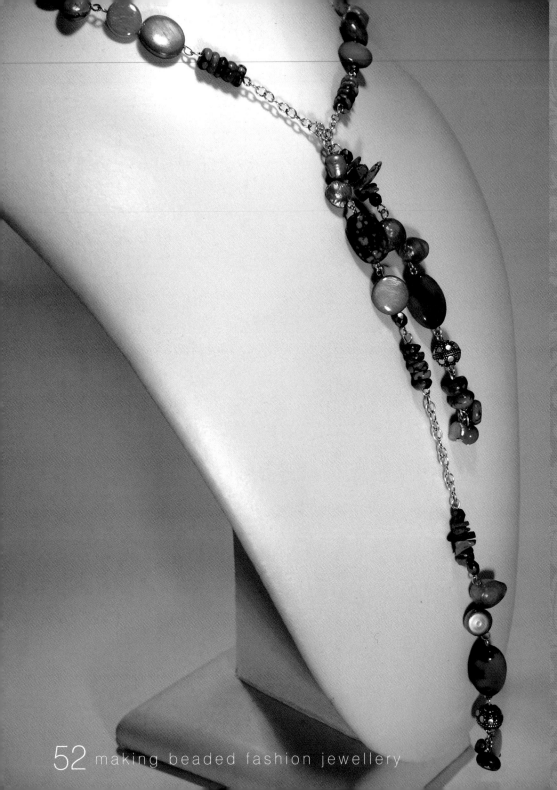

I've chosen to use my birthstone Turquoise to make this lariat, but you can swap the turquoise for your own birthstone or any stone of your choice. Using a birthstone to make a piece of jewellery makes it more personalized and its a great way to make a special birthday present.

*Turquoise beads, chips, pearls, Bali spacer beads, and a huge variety of other semi-precious stones are all available from KernowCraft or Rashbel UK. Bead Reamer's can be purchased from G J Beads, more information on all these stockists can be found on the stockist's pages at the back of the book.

turquoise lariat necklace

YOU WILL NEED

Turquoise chip beads

Turquoise rondelles

Turquoise nugget beads

Silver plated or sterling silver chain

Silver plated or sterling silver charms/tassel

Pearls

Head pins

Eye pins

Czech glass

Mother of pearl discs

Bali Spacer beads

Bead Reamer

step-by-step

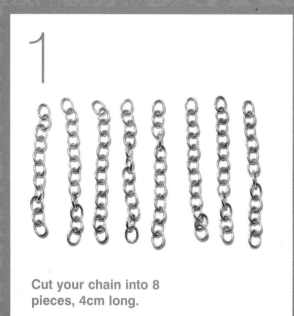

1

Cut your chain into 8 pieces, 4cm long.

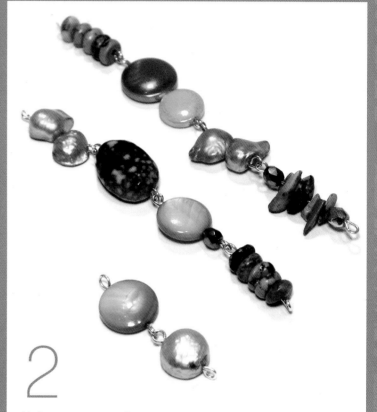

2

Using your eye pins and making a loop at both ends, start making individual sections of beads, using the different types of stone shapes to add variety to this one long piece.

If you find any of your pearls have holes that are too small for the eye pins, try using a bead reamer. (For more information on this handy tool see the tools section at the front of the book.)

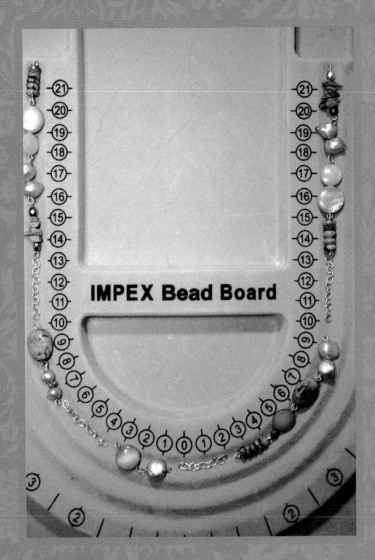

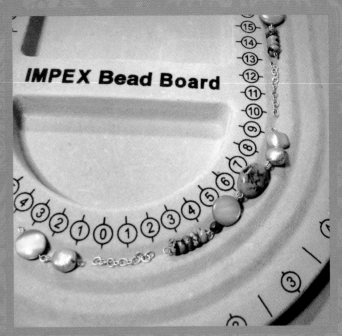

Once you're happy with your layout attach the sections to the lengths of chain by opening your loops.

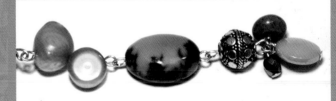

3 Try laying out your sections on a bead board to help you see what sits well together. Your design doesn't have to be symmetrical like mine, why not try experimenting with asymmetry, which works well for this style of necklace.

4 At the ends of the chain use some of your favourite beads, (these will be seen first because they will be at the front of the necklace.) Add drops to this bead using the loop making technique in the basics section.

step-by-step

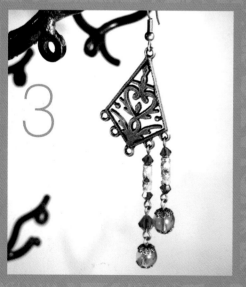

Open the loop on your earring findings and attach the chandelier finding.

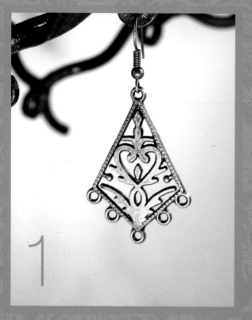

Make beaded links by adding small beads onto eye pins and making a loop at the end, then use two bead caps to jazz up a simple 8mm bead and make it into a hanging drop, by threading it onto a head pin and making a loop. (See Basics section for instructions on making plain loops.)

Now just repeat your design.

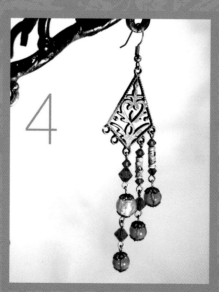

Create different lengths by adding some larger beads to your design.

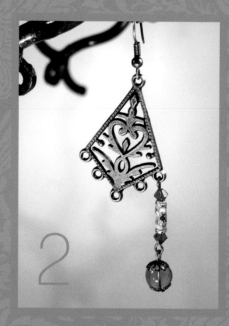

chandelier earrings

YOU WILL NEED

A pair of chandelier earring findings

A pair of earring wires

Head pins

Eye pins

Cloisonné tube beads

4mm Swarovski crystal beads

6mm Swarovski crystal beads

Beads caps

8mm glass beads

8mm silver lined Venetian beads

These fantastic bronze colour findings are available from Regal Crafts; you can find their information on the stockist's pages.

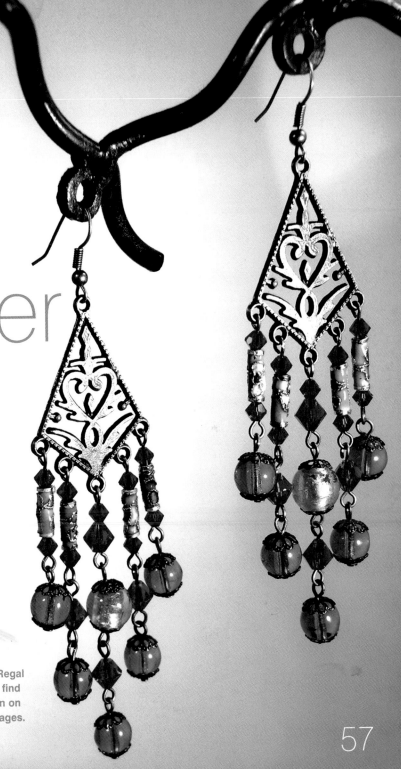

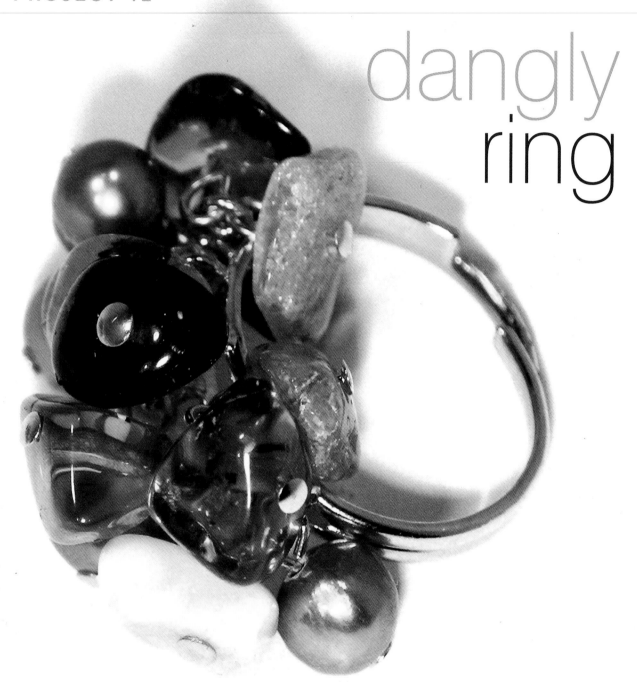

dangly
ring

step-by-step

YOU WILL NEED

Amber chips

Ring finding with loops

Freshwater pearls

Head pins

Adjustable ring finding with loops

* These handy ring findings can be purchased from Bijoux Beads. You can find Amber chips and pearls at Buffy's Beads; their contact information can be found on the stockists pages.

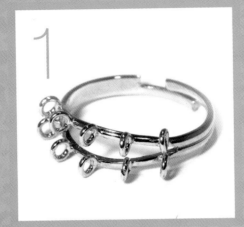

Start by taking an expandable ring finding with soldered loops.

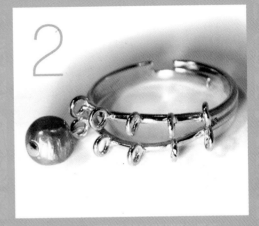

Make a drop by putting a pearl onto a head pin and making a loop. (Check the techniques in the Basics section for a reminder.)

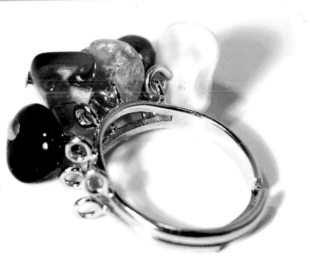

All you need to do now is keep adding more beads and pearls until you are happy that your ring has plenty of dangles, so when you move your hand the bare finding is not exposed.

step-by-step

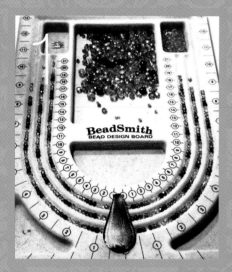

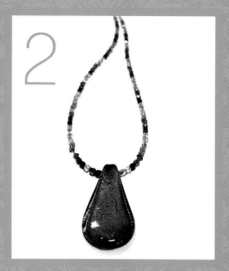

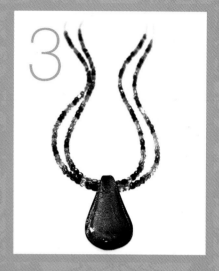

Use your trusty bead board to lay out your design.

Begin by threading beads onto your first strand. When you get to the middle of the length of wire thread through the hanging loop of your pendant.

Repeat the same design on the following two strands of wire and thread them through the pendant hanging loop.

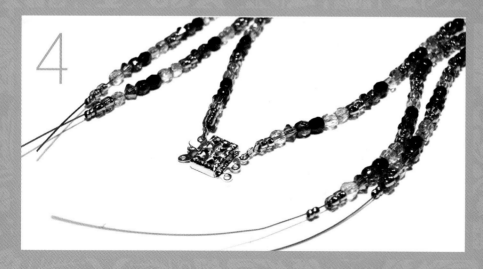

To complete the necklace add two crimps to each end of the three strands. You should have 6 crimps in all. Start from the inside strand and work outwards, one by one to thread these through the clasp and back through the crimps and the beads on the end of the necklace for added strength. At this stage it's easy to rush and drop a strand. Just stay calm and give yourself plenty of time. Focus on one strand at a time, secure it, make sure the beads are right up against the clasp then, crimp it and then go onto the next.

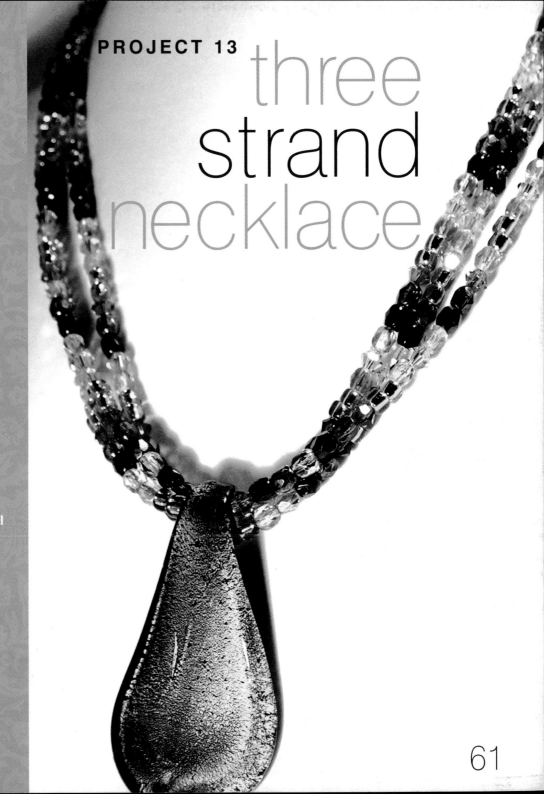

A natural progression from the two strand bracelet, this project looks fantastic and very professional once it's finished. The pattern is up to you, I chose a simple but effective light to dark design.

three strand necklace

YOU WILL NEED

Size 11 seed beads

4mm Swarovski crystals

4mm Czech glass beads

Beading wire

3 strand clasp

Crimps

Crimping pliers

Focal bead with a large loop, I chose a Venetian glass pendant

* You can find a wonderful selection of Venetian glass beads and pendants at www.beadsbyyvonne.co.uk

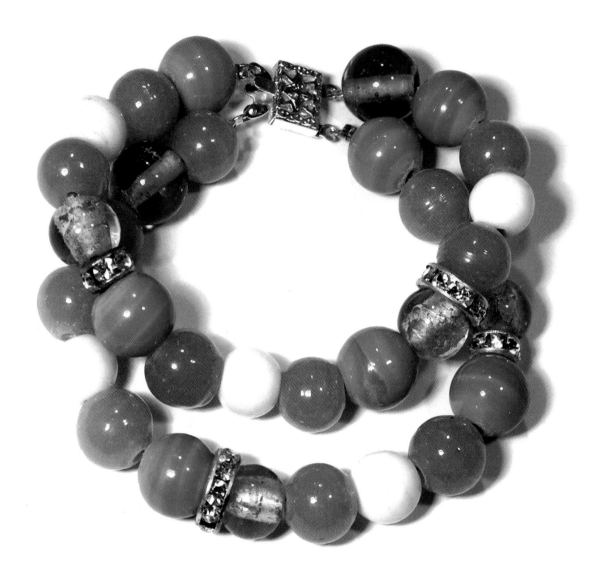

two strand bracelet

step-by-step

Making any multi-strand project may look daunting at first, but once you have made a few of these two strand bracelets you'll be able to use the same techniques to make as many multi-strand pieces as you want! The trick is not to rush and focus on one strand at a time. Once you have secured the first strand you can move onto the next.

YOU WILL NEED

Tape measure

Beading wire

Bead board

2 strand clasp

Crimps

Crimping pliers

Rhinestone rondelles

8mm glass beads

8mm silver foil lined

Venetian glass beads

1 Cut two pieces of beading wire, both the same length that fit your wrist and add an extra 3cm onto each end.

2 Lay out your design on a bead board so you can see how the two strands will look together.

3 Once you're happy with the design put two crimp beads on each end of both strands of beads. Attach the clasp by threading the wire through the loops on each side.

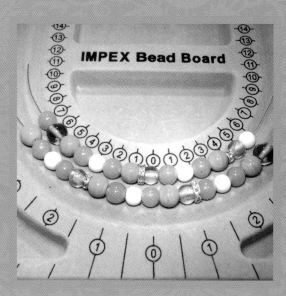

4 Once you're happy with the design put two crimp beads on each end of both strands of beads. Attach the clasp by threading the wire through the loops on each side. Then all you have to do is thread the wire back through the crimp beads on each of the four loose wires you have. Take your time, if you rush you might drop one strand and have to re-thread it. Just concentrate on one strand at a time so you don't mix the strands up.

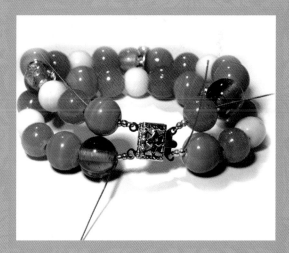

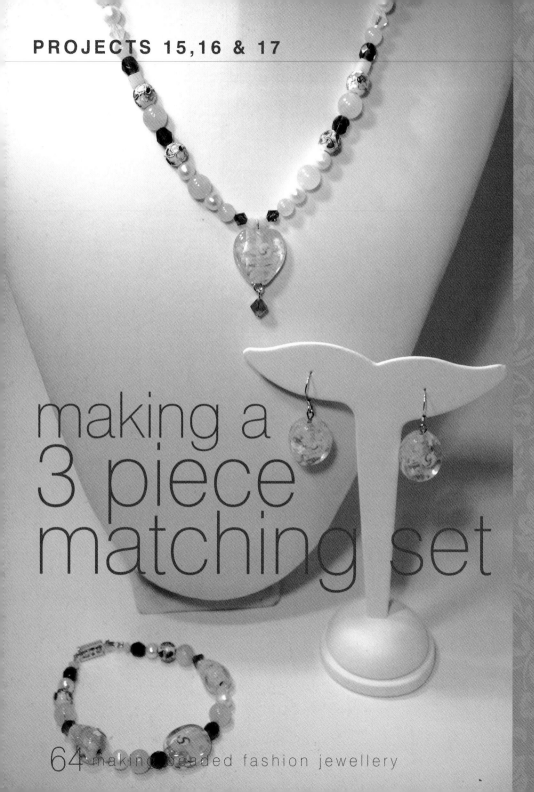

making a 3 piece matching set

YOU WILL NEED

1 pair of earring findings

2 matching single strand clasps

Beading wire

Head pins

Eye pins

Round nose pliers

Wire cutters

Crimp beads

Crimping pliers

6 matching focal beads of your choice (I used Venetian style glass beads)

6mm Swarovski crystals in 3 different colours

6mm Chinese Cloisonné beads

6mm White Freshwater pearls

6mm Czech glass bead

6mm Rose Quartz beads

8mm Rose Quartz beads

to make the necklace

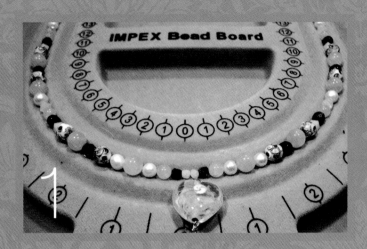

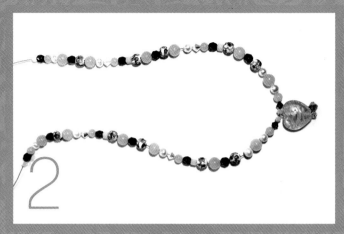

When making a matching set it helps to lay everything out before you start to see how things look. Using a bead board can help you to design your necklace, bracelet and matching earrings before you start putting them together, and at this stage it's easy to swap beads around.

Once you are happy with your design you're ready to put it together. Start by making the pendant for your necklace. Put your favourite focal bead onto an eye pin and make a loop, then attach a pearl or crystal drop onto the bottom loop. (Check the techniques in the Basics section for a reminder.)

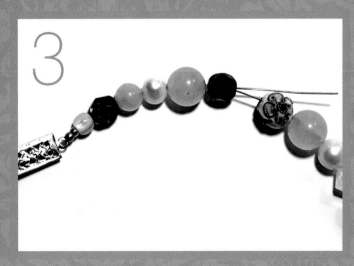

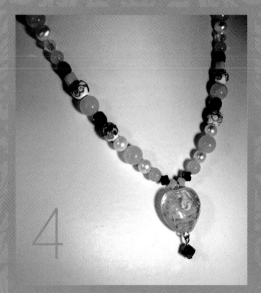

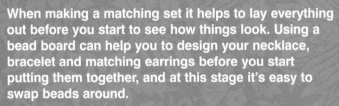

Add two crimps to each end of your necklace and thread the wire back through the crimps and at least three extra beads for security.

Thread through the top loop of the pendant and begin adding your choice of beads.

making the bracelet

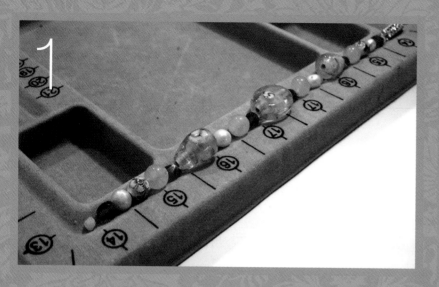

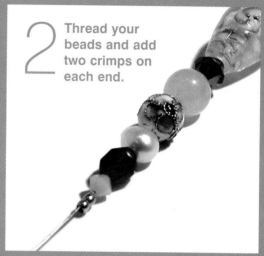

Thread your beads and add two crimps on each end.

Layout your design on the bead board to match necklace. You don't have to repeat the pattern of your necklace but it helps. Cut a length of beading wire to fit your wrist, adding an extra 3cm on each end.

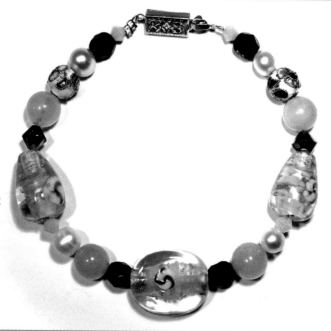

Thread your wire back through the crimps and 3 extra beads. Make sure to crush the crimps and cut off any excess wire.

making the earrings

1

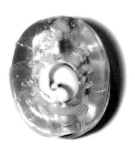

Take your two remaining matching focal beads.

2

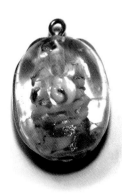

Thread each one onto a head pin and make a loop. (Check the Basics page for a reminder on how.)

3

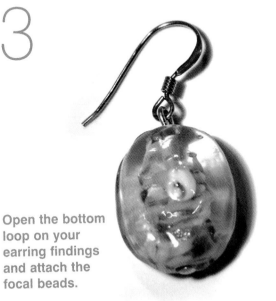

Open the bottom loop on your earring findings and attach the focal beads.

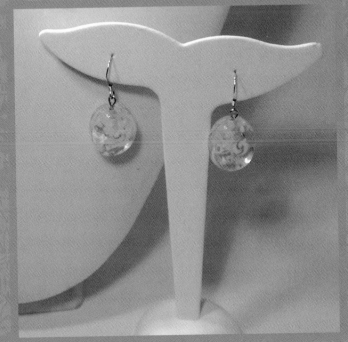

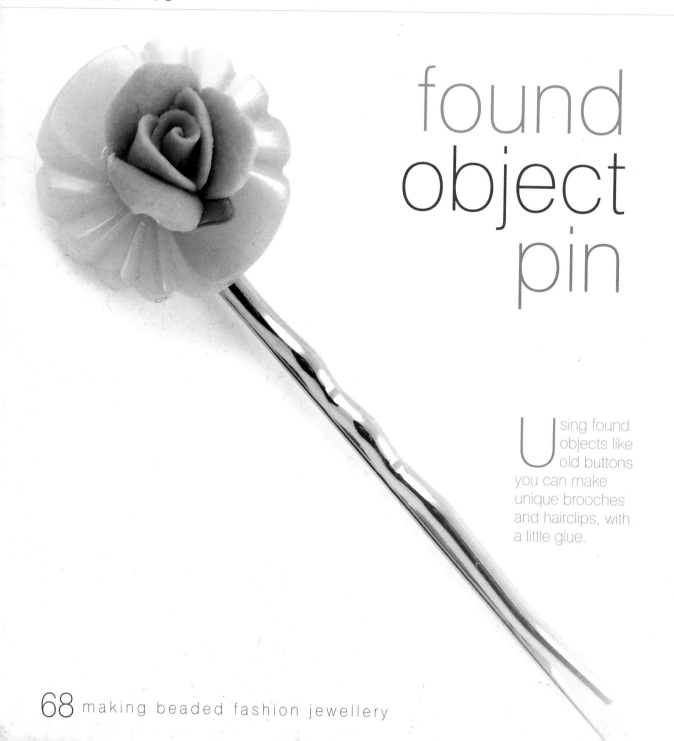

found
object
pin

U sing found
objects like
old buttons
you can make
unique brooches
and hairclips, with
a little glue.

step-by-step

YOU WILL NEED

Old buttons with a flat back (no shank)

Bead cement*

Porcelain flower

Small brooch bar or hair clip with flat pad

* You can buy bead cement from www.beadsbyyvonne.co.uk

1

Select your button and a suitable centrepiece, I chose a porcelain flower.

2

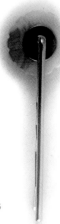

Position the flat pad of the hairclip in the centre of the back of the button, then using the beading cement glue the two pieces together and leave to dry.

3

Dab a little bead cement on the back of the porcelain flower and position it in the centre of the button, covering the holes, then leave to dry.

* Making a brooch pin instead of a hairclip is easy, just glue the brooch bar on instead of the hairclip, and remember to use a button that's large enough to cover the pin itself. You can buy brooch bars from www.jillybeads.co.uk

step-by-step

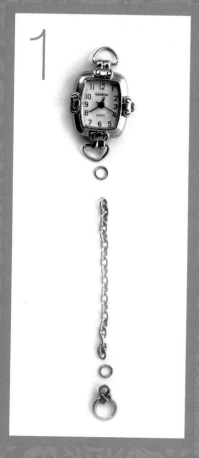

1

The standard bracelet measurement is 17cm, this may be too small/big for you so make sure to measure your wrist. Subtract the length of your chosen watch face from this measurement and that tells you how much chain you will need.

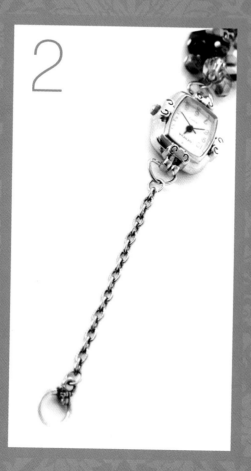

2

Cut your length of chain into two equal sections. Then attach the end to the watch face with a jump ring and attach the other end to one half of the toggle clasp.

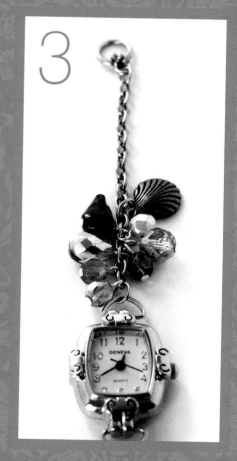

3

Begin to add beads to your length of chain, repeat the order of beads to have an equal blend of colours and shapes, adding your charms last. Then just repeat this with your second piece of chain.

beaded watch strap

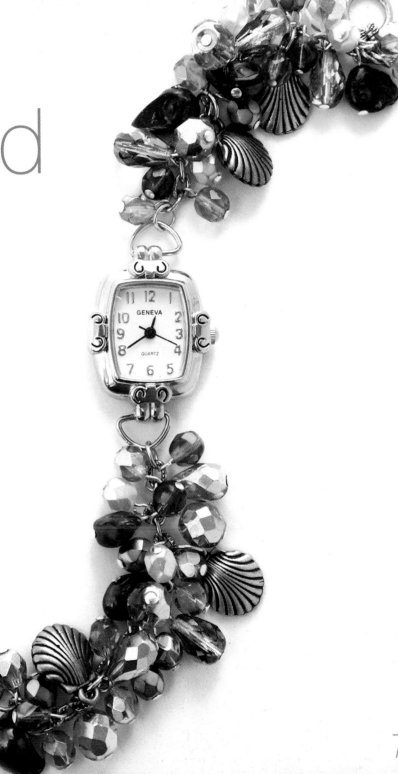

YOU WILL NEED

Chain

Head pins

Charms

6mm Czech glass beads

Jump rings

Toggle clasp

Freshwater pearls

Watch face *

* You can buy watch faces
  from www.jillybeads.co.uk

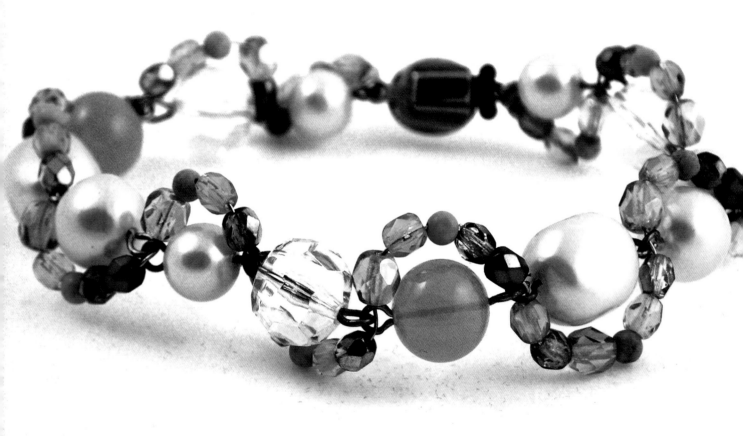

double helix bracelet

YOU WILL NEED

Eye pins

3mm, 4mm, 8mm, 10mm beads in matching colours

8mm, 9mm, 10mm Faux pearls

26 gauge beading wire

Crimps

Toggle clasp

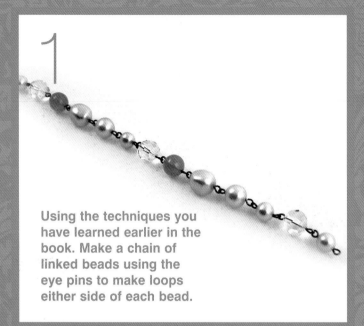

1

Using the techniques you have learned earlier in the book. Make a chain of linked beads using the eye pins to make loops either side of each bead.

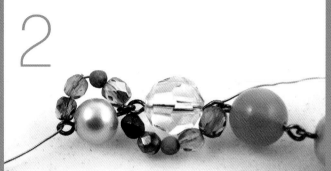

2

Leaving plenty of excess cut a piece of beading wire.

Thread the wire through the first of your beaded links, then start to thread your 3 and 4mm beads, only use enough to fit snugly over the top of the bead, then thread through the next link, this time you'll be going under the bead.

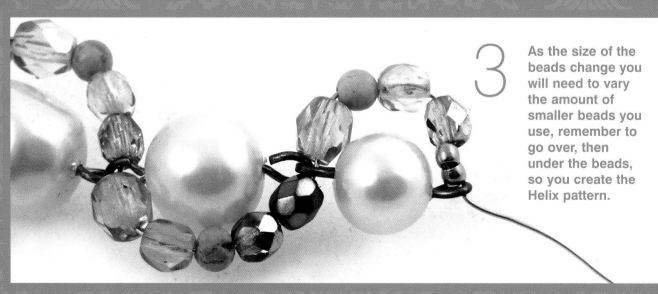

3

As the size of the beads change you will need to vary the amount of smaller beads you use, remember to go over, then under the beads, so you create the Helix pattern.

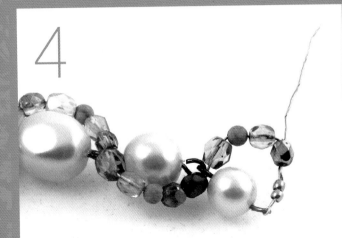

4

Keep shaping the wire with your fingers to mirror the curves of the bead. Pull it tight each time you move onto the next bead so it retains its shape.

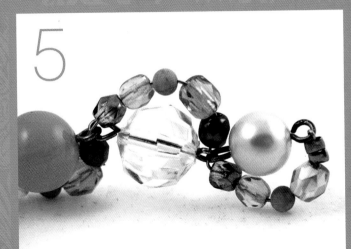

5

When you have reached the end of your beaded chain, and have threaded through each link, add two crimps to your wire.

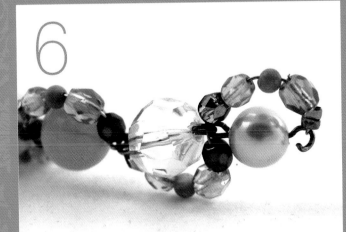

6

Thread the wire through the last link in the chain and back through a couple of beads on the end for added strength. Then crush the crimps, and trim the excess wire.

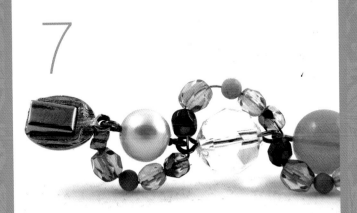

7

Carefully open the last link in the chain to attach the toggle clasp.

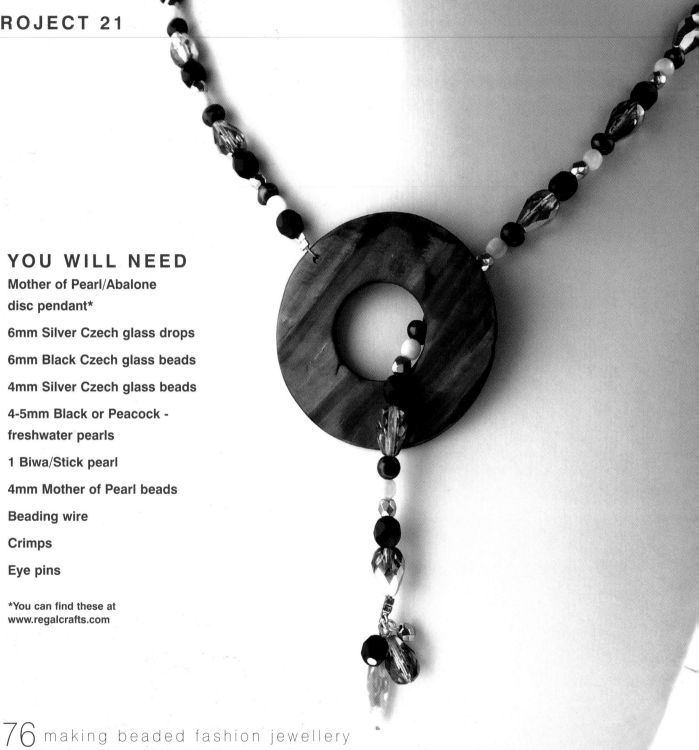

YOU WILL NEED

Mother of Pearl/Abalone disc pendant*

6mm Silver Czech glass drops

6mm Black Czech glass beads

4mm Silver Czech glass beads

4-5mm Black or Peacock - freshwater pearls

1 Biwa/Stick pearl

4mm Mother of Pearl beads

Beading wire

Crimps

Eye pins

*You can find these at www.regalcrafts.com

monochrome disc necklace

step-by-step

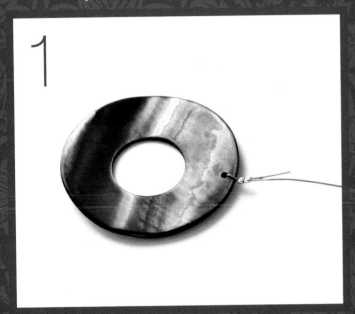

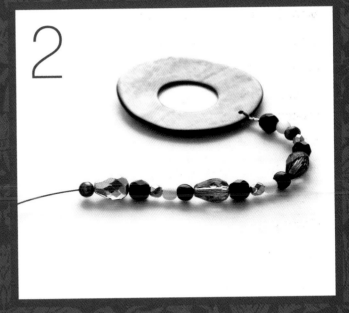

Thread your length of beading wire through the small hole in the disc and add two crimps to your wire, thread back through the crimps and crush them.

Now you can start threading your beads. The repeating pattern is key to the design of this necklace so choose an order to thread the beads on and stick to it, or just copy mine.

step-by-step

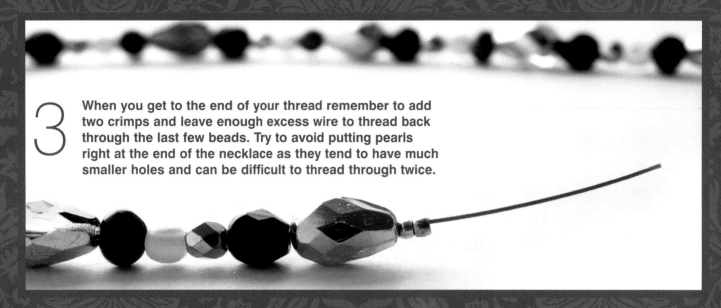

3 When you get to the end of your thread remember to add two crimps and leave enough excess wire to thread back through the last few beads. Try to avoid putting pearls right at the end of the necklace as they tend to have much smaller holes and can be difficult to thread through twice.

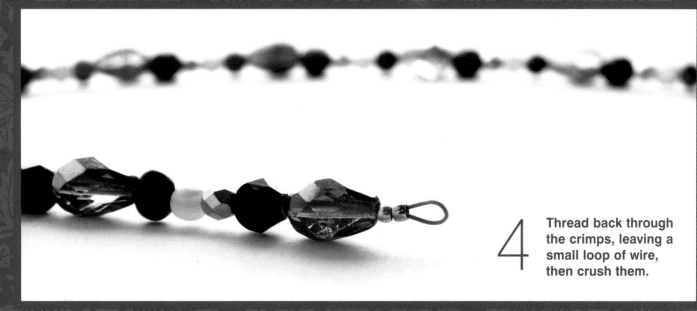

4 Thread back through the crimps, leaving a small loop of wire, then crush them.

5

Make the Biwa pearl and some of the other beads you used in the necklace drops and dangles, and put them together to make a small tassel. To add them to the necklace simply open the top loop of the Biwa Pearl drop and attach to wire loop.

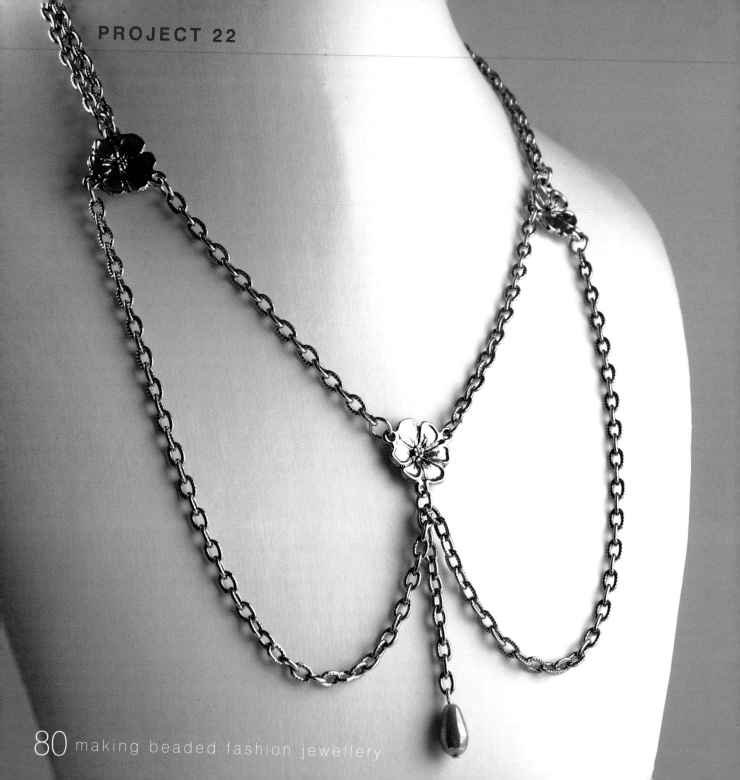

chain necklace

step-by-step

1

Cut four lengths of chain into equal 10cm parts. These will make up the back of your necklace. Attach a jump ring to each end, two pieces will be attached to the either side of the clasp.

YOU WILL NEED

Chain

Jump rings

3 loop connectors

6mm drop bead

Head pin

Spring ring clasp

Neck bust

2

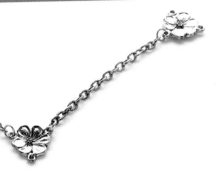

For the front of your necklace you will need another four lengths of chain, but this time of two different lengths, 6cm and 16cm.
   Put jump rings on each end of the 6cm chain pieces and open these to attach to the loops of your connectors.

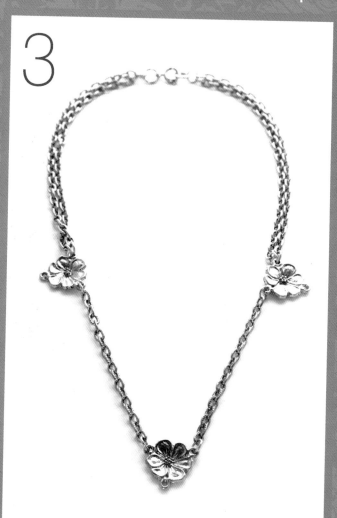

3

One by one open the four jump rings on your 10cm pieces of chain, to connect the back of the necklace to the front.

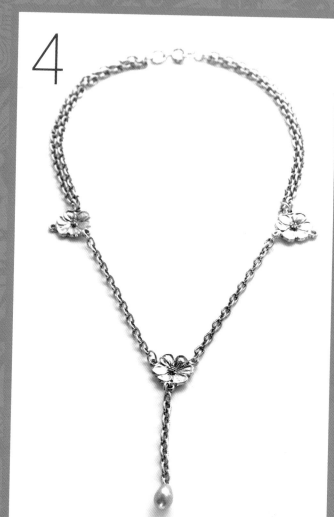

4

Cut a piece of chain 3.5cm long, attach the drop to this and hang it from the centre connector by a jump ring.

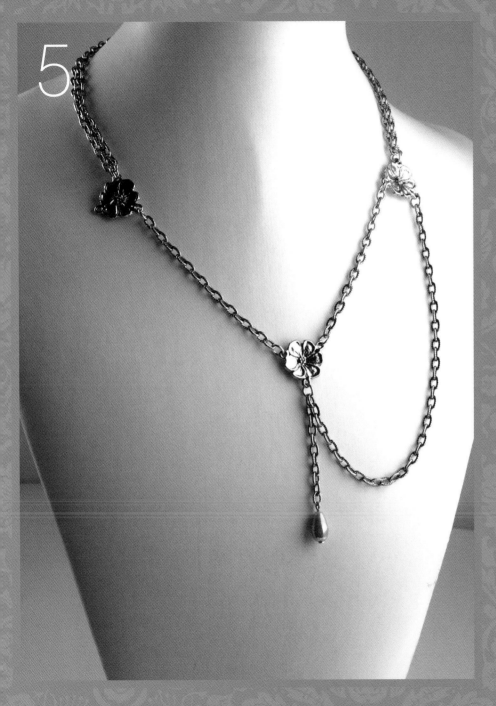

5

So that you can see how the chain hangs, it is very useful to use a neck bust for this next step.

Drape the 16cm section of chain across the bust, and using jump rings link it to the connector on the right hand side and then down to the centre connector. You already have a jump ring here from the centre drop, so attach it to this jump ring. Just repeat this step for the left hand side.

bead society
of great britain

The Bead Society of Great Britain, (formed in September 1989), is a subscription-based, non-profit making, non-commercial venture run by a permanent team who work voluntarily. The Society is open to all those who have an appreciation, either private or professional, of beads ancient and modern, of all shapes, sizes, materials and colours; their techniques of manufacture, and their application. The Society numbers among its members: private collectors, researchers, dealers, jewellery makers, bead embroiderers, beadwork weavers, makers of beads, and many others - so there's a place for everyone.

The Bead Society has a newsletter which is an illustrated colour journal of bead related articles, projects, events and information etc., and of usually 32 pages, which is sent to all members four times a year.

The Bead Society of Great Britain holds an annual bead fair in Harrow usually on the first Sunday in October every year. If you like your beads it's an event well worth a visit, you can buy everything you'll ever need to bead under one roof, whether you want beads, jewellery, gemstones, findings, tools or books. There are also workshops, talks and usually a visit to see a collection/museum, most free to members.

Admission is free to members and £2.00 for non members.

For membership inquiries please contact:
Honorary Secretary
Dr Carole Morris
1 Casburn Lane, Burwell
Cambs, CB25 0ED
– please send SSAE
for membership details

For more information,
membership forms and details
of this year's fair please see:
www.beadsociety.freeserve.co.uk

UK bead stockists

CENTRAL LONDON

London Bead Co
339 Kentish Town Road
NW5 2TJ
www.londonbeadco.co.uk
Tel: 0870 203 2323/202 8007

The Bead Shop
21a Tower Street
Covent Garden
London
WC2H 9NS
www.beadshop.co.uk
Tel: 020 7240 0931

Bead Aura
3 Neal's Yard
Covent Garden
WC2H 9DP
Tel: 020 7836 3002

Buffy's Beads
2.3 Kingly Court
Kingly Street
London
W1B 5PW
www.buffysbeads.com
Tel: 020 7494 2323

Creative Beadcraft
20 Beak Street
London
W1F 9RE
www.creativebeadcraft.co.uk
Tel: 020 7629 9964

Anita's Beads
51 Burnthwaite Road
Fulham
London
SW6 5BQ
Tel: 020 7385 5952

Creative Beadcraft
(formerly Ells & Farrier)
20 Beak Street
London
W1F 9RE
www.creativebeadcraft.co.uk
020 7629 9964

Rashbel
24-28 Hatton Wall
London
EC1N 8JH
www.rashbel.com
Tel: 020 7831 5646

Grifoni Ltd
20 Denbigh Road
West Ealing
London
W13 8QB
www.grifoni.co.uk
Tel: 020 8810 4418

GREATER LONDON

Sylvia Joyce Gems
The Treasury
2 Barters Walk
Pinner
Middlesex
HA5 5LU
Tel: 020 8866 3533

Czech Beads
2 St Catherine's Rd
Ruislip
Middlesex
HA4 7RU
www.czechbeads.co.uk
Tel: 0788 171 6484

Elle-Art Mosaic and Beads
46 Victoria Rd
Ruislip
Middlesex
HA4 0AG
www.elle-art.co.uk
Tel: 01895 633 528

Charisma Beads
25 Churchyard
Hitchin
Hertfordshire
SG5 1HP
www.charismabeads.co.uk
Tel: 01462 454 054

BEDFORDSHIRE

Regal Crafts
269 Meadow Way
Leighton Buzzard
Bedfordshire
LU5 4JP
www.regalcrafts.com

Mr Bead
1 The Firs
Wigmore Lane
Luton
Bedfordshire
LU2 8AA
www.mrbead.com
Tel: 0870 132 9414

BIRMINGHAM

Beadgems
P.O. Box 12310
Birmingham
West Midlands
B13 3AE
www.beadgems.com
Tel: 0845 123 2743

BRISTOL

Grove Beads
3 Grove Park
Brislington
Bristol
BS4 3LG
www.grovebeads.co.uk

CAMBRIDGESHIRE

The Rocking Rabbit Bead Shop
7 The Green
Haddenham
Ely
CB6 3TA
www.rockingrabbit.co.uk
Tel: 0870 606 1588

K & M Beadshop
18 Pelham Close
Cottenham
Cambridge
CB4 8TY
www.kandmbeadshop.com
Tel: 07739 801 932

Spangles (Int)
1 Casburn Lane
Burwell
Cambridge
CB5 0ED
www.spangles4beads.co.uk

CHESHIRE

Manchester Minerals

Georges Road
Stockport
Cheshire
SK4 1DP
www.manchesterminerals.co.uk
Tel: 0161 480 5095

BeadAddict.co.uk

8 Charter Close
Sale
Cheshire
M33 6LF
www.beadaddict.co.uk
Tel: 0161 973 1945

The Bead Shop

20 Frodsham Street
Chester
Cheshire
CH1 3JL
www.the-beadshop.co.uk
Tel: 01244 409 457

21st Century Beads

Craft Workshops
South Pier Road
Ellesmere Port
South Wirral
Cheshire
CH65 4FW
www.beadmaster.com
Tel: 0151 356 4444

CORNWALL

Chapel Crafts & Beads

1 Chapel Terrace
Porthleven
Helston
Cornwall
TR13 9HS
Tel: 01326 565 733

Kernowcraft Rocks & Gems Ltd

Bolingey
Perranporth
Cornwall
TR6 0DH
www.kernowcraft.com
Tel: 01872 573 888

GJ Beads

Unit 1 Court Arcade
The Wharf
St Ives
Cornwall
TR26 1LG
www.gjbeads.co.uk
Tel: 01736 751 070

Meerkat Beads

41b Killigrew Street
Falmouth
Cornwall
TR11 3PW
www.meerkatbeads.co.uk
Tel: 01326 212 554

DERBYSHIRE

Empirical Praxis Ltd

27 Abbeyhill
Chesterfield
Derbyshire
S42 7JL
www.epbeads.co.uk
Tel: 01246 556 988

DEVONSHIRE

Bunyip Beads & Buttons

Units 7-10
McCoys Arcade
Fore Street
Exeter
Devon
EX4 3AN
www.bunyip.myzen.co.uk
Tel: 01392 437 377

DORSET

Parkers Jewellery at
The Bead 'n' Glass Studio

The Courtyard Craft Centre
Huntick Road
Lychett Minster
Poole
Dorset
BH16 6BA
www.parkersjewellery.co.uk
Tel: 01202 622 040

Bijoux Beads

Swans Yard
High Street
Shaftsbury
Dorset
SP7 8JQ
www.bijouxbeads.co.uk
Tel: 01225 482 024

Stitch 'n' Craft

Swan's Yard
High St
Shaftsbury
Dorset
SP7 8JQ
www.stitchncraft.co.uk
Tel: 01747 852 500

ESSEX

Pandorion

29 East Hill
Colchester
Essex
CO1 2QX
www.pandorion.co.uk
Tel: 01206 868 623

Novacraft

221 London Road
Rayleigh
Essex
SS6 9DN
www.littlebeader.com/novacraftuk.htm
Tel: 01268 786 667

JRM Beads, Ltd. (Beadworks)

16 Redbridge Enterprise Centre
Thompson Close
Ilford
Essex
IG1 1TY
www.beadworks.co.uk
Tel: 020 8553 3240

Ideas Unlimited

Cymru Fach
17 Wick Farm Road
St Lawrence Bay
Southminster
Essex
CM0 7PF
www.ideas-un-limited.co.uk
Tel: 01621 778 804

Bee Jewelled

Unit 9
Station Road
Nr Halstead
Sible Hedingham
Essex
C09 3PY
www.beejewelled.com
Tel: 01787 463 258

HAMPSHIRE

Kingfisher Beads

81 Harold Road
Stubbington
Fareham
Hampshire
P014 2QP
www.kingfisherbeads.co.uk

World of Beads

1 Stonemason's Court
Parchment Street
Winchester
Hampshire
S023 8AT
www.worldofbeads.co.uk
Tel: 01962 861 255

HEREFORDSHIRE
Beads-in-Abundance
Unit 4
Capuchin Yard
Church Street
Hereford
Herefordshire
HR1 2LR
www.beadsinabundance.com
Tel: 01432 357 230

KENT
The Bead Garden
2 Fairey Avenue
Hayes
Kent
UB3 4NY
www.thebead-garden.com

LANCASHIRE
JillyBeads
1 Anstable Road
Morecambe
Lancashire
LA4 6TG
www.jillybeads.co.uk
Tel: 01524 412 728

Bead Shop
Afflecks Palace
52 Church Street
Manchester
Lancashire
M4 1PW
Tel: 0161 833 9950

LEICESTERSHIRE
Beads for Benders Ltd
Castle View Farm
Hickling Lane
Long Clawson
Leicestershire
LE14 4NW
www.beadsforbeaders.com
Tel: 01664 822 389

LINCOLNSHIRE
The Bead Gallery
19 Clasketgate
Lincoln
Lincolnshire
LN2 1JJ
Tel: 01522 525 080

NORTHAMPTONSHIRE
International Craft
Unit 4
The Empire Centre
Imperial Way
Watford
Northamptonshire
WD24 4YH
www.internationalcraft.com
Tel: 01923 235 336

NOTTINGHAMSHIRE
Beads by Yvonne
232 Haydn Road
Sherwood
Nottingham
Nottinghamshire
NG5 2LG
www.beadsbyyvonne.co.uk
Tel: 0115 962 2400

The Bead Shop
(Nottingham) Ltd
7 Market Street
Nottingham
Nottinghamshire
NG1 6HY
www.mailorder-beads.co.uk
Tel: 0115 958 8899

OXFORDSHIRE

Glass and Stone

3 Victoria Cross Gallery

Rolls Court

The Market Place

Wantage

Oxfordshire

OX12 9AE

www.glassandstone.co.uk

Tel: 01235 772 074

SHROPSHIRE

Jules Gems Ltd

Unit A

GDS Building

Lancaster Road

Shrewsbury

SY1 3LG

www.julesgems.com

Tel: 0845 123 5828

SOMERSET

Bijoux Beads

Elton House

2 Abbey Street

Bath

BA1 1NN

www.bijouxbeads.co.uk

Tel: 01225 482 024

STAFFORDSHIRE

The Spellbound Bead Company

45 Tamworth Street

Staffordshire

WS13 6JW

www.spellboundbead.co.uk

Tel: 01543 417 650

Make Jewellery

Silvar Design

111 High Street

Wolstanton

Newcastle under Lyme

ST5 0EP

www.makejewellery.co.uk

SURREY

Emma Ralph

E J R Beads

81 Woodcote

Grove Road

Coulsdon

Surrey

CR5 2AL

www.ejrbeads.co.uk

SUSSEX

Beads Unlimited

The Brighton Bead Shop

21 Sydney St

Brighton

BN1 4EN

www.beadsunlimited.co.uk

Tel: 01273 675 077

Mad About Beads

Glyndale - St. Mary's Lane

Ticehurst

Wadhurst

East Sussex

TN5 7AX

www.madaboutbeads.com

TYNE AND WEAR

Rosarama Beadcraft

2 Beech Grove Terrace

Crawcrook

Ryton

Gateshead

Tyne and Wear

NE40 4LZ

Cottonwood Creations

21 Cottonwood

Houghton Le Spring

Tyne and Wear

DH4 7TA

YORKSHIRE

Yum Yum Beads Ltd
3 Thornton's Arcade
Leeds
West Yorkshire
LS21 6LQ
www.yumyumbeads.co.uk
Tel: 0113 244 2888

Magpie Jewellery
P.O. Box 3926
Sheffield
S5 5AF
South Yorkshire
www.magpiejewellery.co.uk
Tel: 07910 026 920

Constellation Beads
The Studio
15 St Nicholas Drive
Richmond
North Yorkshire
DL10 7DY
www.constellationbeads.co.uk
Tel: 01748 826 552

Beads by Design
4 Nunnery Walk
South Cave
Brough
East Yorkshire
HU15 2JA
www.beadsbydesign.co.uk
Tel: 01430 471 007

WALES

Jewel Box International
99 Bowen Court
St. Asaph Business Park
St. Asaph
Denbighshire
LL17 0JE
www.jewelboxinternational.com
0870 770 4968

INTERNATIONAL STOCKISTS

Rio Grande
www.riogrande.com
Tel: 1 800 545 6566

Fire Mountain Gems
www.firemountaingems.com
Tel: 1 800 355 2137

acknowledgements

Completing this book would not have been possible without the help of the following people. I'd like to thank my understanding publisher Susan James at A&C Black. My cousins, Ben Usiskin for his encouragement and Dan Usiskin for his fabulous photography and my long suffering partner Arash Aframian, who lets me drag him to bead shops wherever we go.

Many bead shops across the UK have shown their support for this book by contributing samples. I would especially like to thank, lampwork bead artist Emma Ralph who generously made me some fabulous beads especially for this book. Carole Morris of the Bead Society of Great Britain. Vivian at Beads by Yvonne, Mark at Regal Crafts, Dawn at Bjoux Beads, Jill at GJ'S beads and the lovely people at Buffy's Beads, and Meerkat Beads.

index